I0505514

HERBAL MEDICINE FOR EVERYONE

THE BEGINNER'S GUIDE TO HEALING COMMON ILLNESSES WITH 20 MEDICINAL HERBS

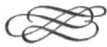

SERENA DAY

SEIZE THE DAY PUBLISHING

CONTENTS

© **Copyright 2020 - All rights reserved.**

The contents of this book may not be reproduced, duplicated, or transmitted without direct written permission from the author.

Under no circumstances will any legal responsibility or blame be held against the publisher for any reparation, damages, or monetary loss due to the information herein, either directly or indirectly.

Legal Notice:

You cannot amend, distribute, sell, use, quote, or paraphrase any part of the content within this book without the consent of the author.

Disclaimer Notice:

Please note the information contained within this document is for educational and entertainment purposes only. No warranties of any kind are expressed or implied. Readers acknowledge that the author is not engaging in the rendering of legal, financial, medical, or professional advice. Please consult a licensed professional before attempting any techniques outlined in this book.

By reading this document, the reader agrees that under no circumstances is the author responsible for any losses, direct or indirect, which are incurred as a result of the use of the information contained within this document, including, but not limited to, —errors, omissions, or inaccuracies.

INTRODUCTION

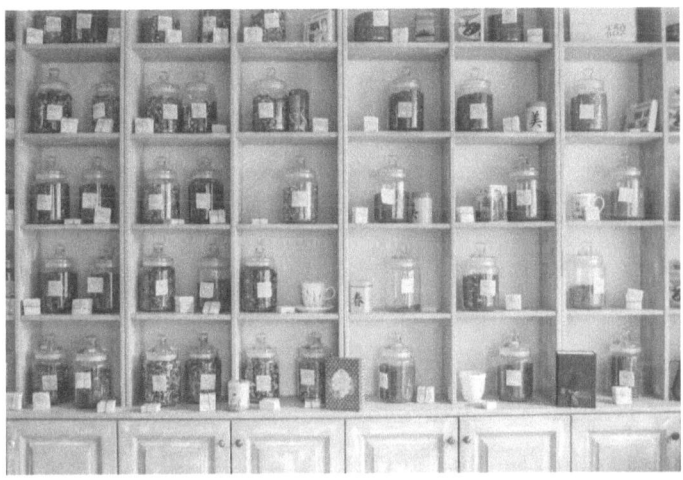

Thank you so much for your decision to take the first step into natural healing and herbalism by getting your hands on a copy of "Herbal Medicine for Everyone."

It can't be denied that there are a million guides and handbooks out there based on the topic of herbalism and medicinal healing. Deciding which one is a good fit can be extremely overwhelming. Fortunately, if you are reading this right now I would like to assure you that you've made the right choice. You are just a few easy steps away from harnessing the power of herbal medicine to alleviate common illnesses.

With the training and guidance provided in this handbook you'll be ready to impress friends and family creating natural and organic cures to illnesses they would have otherwise suffered more from or taken harmful medicines to alleviate.

'Herbal Medicine for Everyone' highlights effective herbs and homemade remedies that assist in the body's natural ability to fight off infections and ultimately cure itself of the common illnesses that plague us frequently.

Nature has always been there for us, long before disinfectants, painkillers, antibiotics, and other commercially produced products were developed. Herbs were steeped to make teas and mixed into poultices.

Herbs have also been used to make tinctures and ointments. They have been expertly used to cure illness for centuries. Natural remedies can treat everything from pain to infections. Amazingly enough, we can find much of what we need growing all around us.

Plants and herbs can be used to create extremely effective medicines, provided they are used correctly. Another major benefit is the fact that most commonly used medicinal herbs are not expensive, especially if you grow them yourself.

This guide will introduce you to the basic principles of growing and making your own herbal remedies and provide valuable recipes to get you started.

You will learn why you should turn to herbal medicine, how to grow and make your own remedies, the most popular herbs used in medicines, and recipes for common ailments.

An Herbal Medicine Orientation will show you what you need to know when it comes to purchasing, making, and using herbal medicine in an effective manner.

A Highly Effective Herbal Overview will teach you about 20 different healing herbs and how to select them appropriately for use in potions and balms.

A Beginner's Guide to Herbalist Healing will

instruct you on 20+ herbal remedies for common ailments provides. It will guide you with step-by-step instructions on how to make each herbal medicine and how to use each medicine effectively.

If you are looking for a new way to heal yourself, a natural way to reduce your pharmaceutical bills or an opportunity to finally cut out all of those unwanted trips to the doctor.

This guide will put you well on your way to becoming a self-taught herbalist and medicinal healer.

PART I
HERBAL MEDICINE – THE BASICS

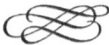

Some people turn their noses up at herbal medicine. They simply don't believe in the healing power of mother nature.

Just as herbs and plants come from nature, so do we.

So, why wouldn't the earth have evolved in a way to provide us with everything we could possibly need? While pharmaceuticals often treat the symptoms of disease, herbal medicine has the power to cure illness in the body.

Not everyone realizes that many of the pharmaceuticals they buy are derived from plants; aspirin, for example, comes from willow bark, while codeine is derived from poppies.

In the next few chapters, you will learn about the benefits of using herbal remedies, some of the methods used, and the tools and equipment you need, most of which you already have in your home.

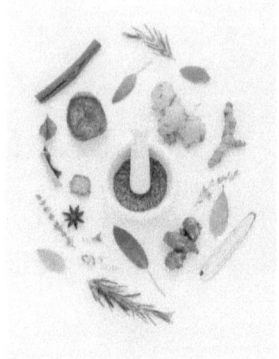

WHAT IS HERBAL MEDICINE?

Herbal medicine is one of the oldest forms of healing and is often called herbalism, phyto-medicine, or botanical medicine. It is the method by which herbs are used for their therapeutic or medicinal value.

Much of what we know about herbal medicine is what has passed down through the generations. Often, because it hasn't been developed using modern scientific methods, it is brushed to one side by Western experts as being alternative medicine. It might surprise many of you to learn that modern medicine uses many of the herbal and plant-based compounds as their basis.

Drugs we use today used to be used as herbal medicines – aspiring, opium, digitalin, and quinine, for example. More than 100 active plant-based compounds are used in today's medicines, and more than 80% of those have a positive correlation with traditional herbal uses of the plants.

Aspirin comes from willow bark, and many parts of the world use it as one of the most effective forms of pain relief.

Across Europe, herbal medicines are popular and can often be found for sale alongside prescription drugs.

It is also so popular in India that the government created the National Medicine Plants Board as a way of overseeing the herbal medicines area.

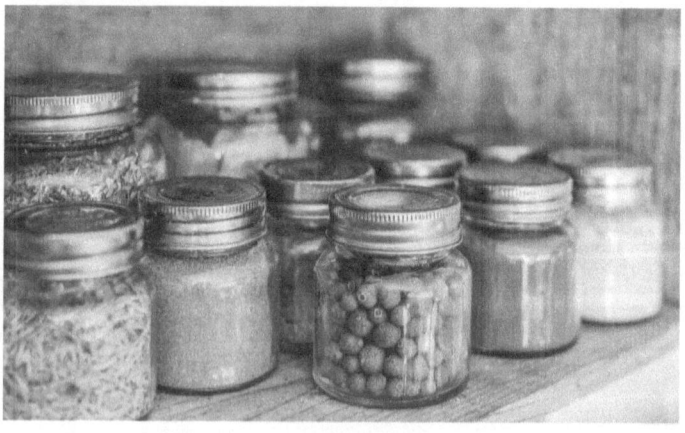

As time passes, more and more people are turning back time and reverting to herbal remedies rather than prescription and over-the-counter medications.

The more you learn about how to use herbal medicine and, more importantly, how to prepare your own safely, the more control you have over your well-being.

NATURE'S ABUNDANT MEDICINE

Herbal medicine can be used to solve quite a few common conditions, sometimes more effectively than modern pharmaceuticals, but without the side effects.

Natural medicines can also help improve your digestive system, boost your immune system and your circulatory system all at the same time.

The multisystemic effect can help eliminate the requirement for several pharmaceuticals, along with the side effects and potential interactions between them.

Herbs are easily accessible to anyone and, even if you opt to buy herbal formulas rather than growing your own, they are still cheaper and safer than many comparable pharmaceuticals. Health care is rising in cost, and, in some parts of the world, it simply isn't affordable to any but a few, and it is in those places where herbal medicines come into their own.

Learning about healing herbs and how to use them will help you to stay healthy naturally, but what are healing herbs?

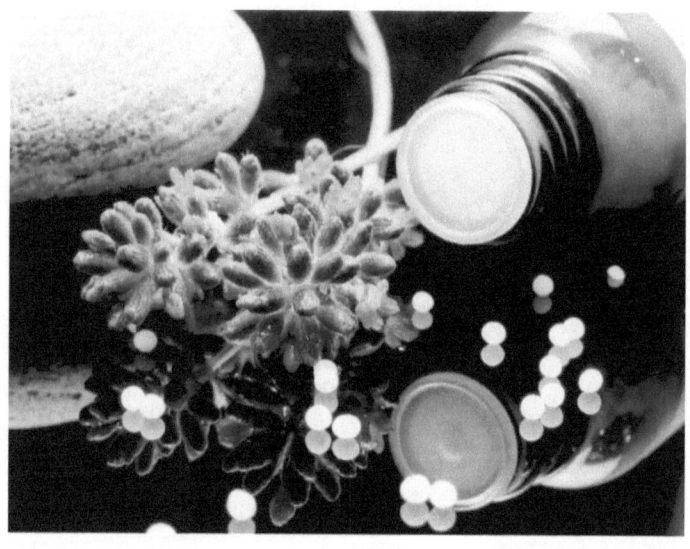

Botanically speaking, an herb is defined as a plant that has leaves and stems that wither and fall off every year.

Biennial and perennial herbs grow a root system that survives while the leaves and stems die off. Annual herbs grow yearly if you plant the seeds or the plant spreads its own seeds.

Typically, an herb is a plant that we can use for food, flavoring, medicine, or fragrance.

Still, as far as herbal medicine goes, the term 'herb' is used rather loosely – not all the plants referred to as herbs for herbal medicine are actually herbs.

Some herbal preparations are ingested, some inhaled, some applied topically, and some can be used in more than one way.

While it isn't always clear to scientists which part of a plant treats ore eliminates symptoms, we do know that entire herbs have components that work together, producing an overall benefit.

Why Use Herbal Medicine?

Not everyone is happy about using herbal medicines, and some don't believe they work.

If you use conventional medicines to treat an ailment or condition, then it's very likely you will be skeptical about swapping to herbal remedies.

Medicinal herbs are full of chemical compounds that offer plenty of therapeutic benefits. Take the native Andeans, for example. Their go-to medicinal plant is the whole coca leaf, no matter what the ailment is.

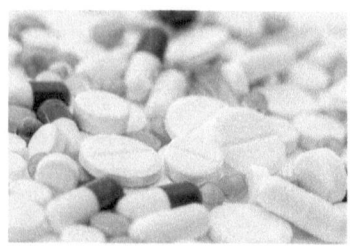

When researchers looked into it, they discovered that the coca plant has 14 different bioactive alkaloids; when the leaf is ingested, digestive tract receptors bind to the alkaloids needed by the body at that time.

Herbal medicine is not about shunning scientific facts, but it also isn't about magic. It's about using a safe, time-tested, evidence-based alternative to treat common ailments.

Many people who take pharmaceuticals suffer, either with bad side effects or interactions between drugs. Around a third of the US population use herbal remedies and most of them have no ill effects whatsoever.

It is a noninvasive, natural way that works with and not against your body. It helps the body build up its natural defenses so long as it is used properly.

And most herbal remedies have been found to have little to no interaction with drugs, nor do they cause toxicity. Rather, they protect the body and help detoxify it at the same time.

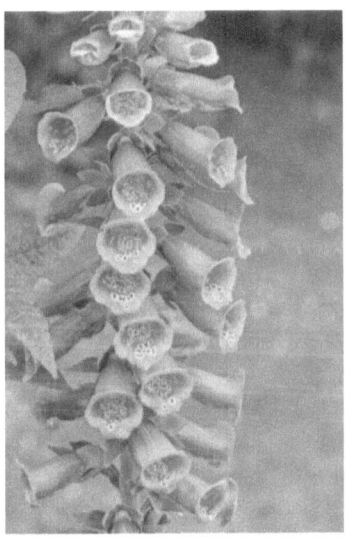

Look at some of the most toxic of pharmaceutical drugs; many of them contain powerful herbal extracts but use those same herbs in the wrong way as herbal medicine, and they can be dangerous.

Take digitalis, for example, the foxglove plant. It produces digitoxin, which is used for heart conditions and taken properly, is incredibly powerful. However, its therapeutic index is narrow, and the wrong dose could be fatal.

AN HERBALIST THAT GROWS HERBS

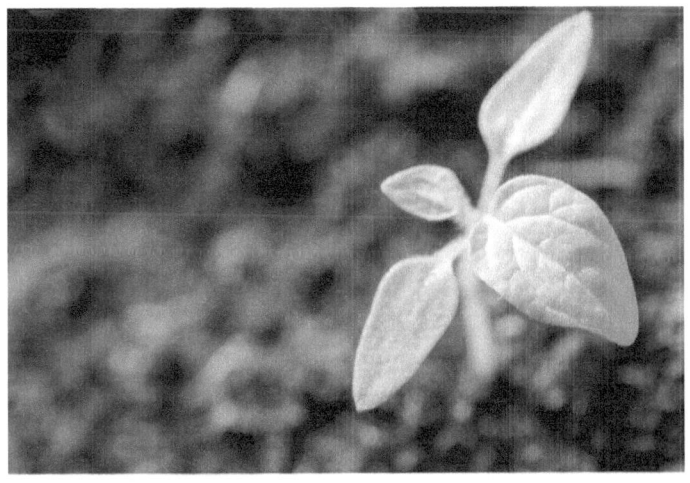

There is every chance that you opted for this book because you are interested in herbal remedies, or you want a safer, more natural way to treat a common ailment.

No matter what your reasoning, there are some important considerations before you begin.

First, think about the ailments you want to treat and base your work on that. Start slowly; don't overwhelm yourself.

You will find some recipes later on for herbal medicines, just make sure you follow the instructions carefully. And, unless indicated that you could do otherwise, only use one remedy at a time.

You will also need certain tools, which we'll be discussing shortly.

One thing you must watch out for are adverts for herbal remedies that claim you will lose a lot of weight fast or those that say they can cure serious diseases.

These are untrue claims, and the remedy may, if you are lucky, do nothing. Otherwise, it could cause you serious problems that require medical intervention to put right.

Perhaps the first place you should start is by growing your own herb garden and getting it set up – in the next part, I'll be telling you of 20 of the most popular and easiest herbs to grow.

Herbal Remedy Considerations

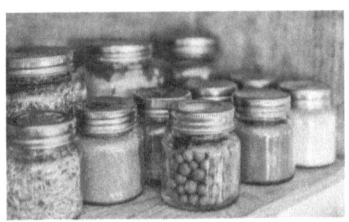

Making an herbal remedy is no different from following a recipe for a new dish.

The right ingredients in the right quantities and combined the right way come together to produce the perfect herbal remedy, the same way as a new dinner dish does.

In many cases, you need only a few tools to pull together a range of useful remedies but, while I will be providing tips on how to prepare plants, but this isn't the main focus of my guide.

I would encourage you to seek additional information elsewhere if preparing plants becomes a passion and particular interest to you.

In the next section I will provide readers with some tricks and tips when it comes to making herbal medicines.

Tips for Making Herbal Medicines

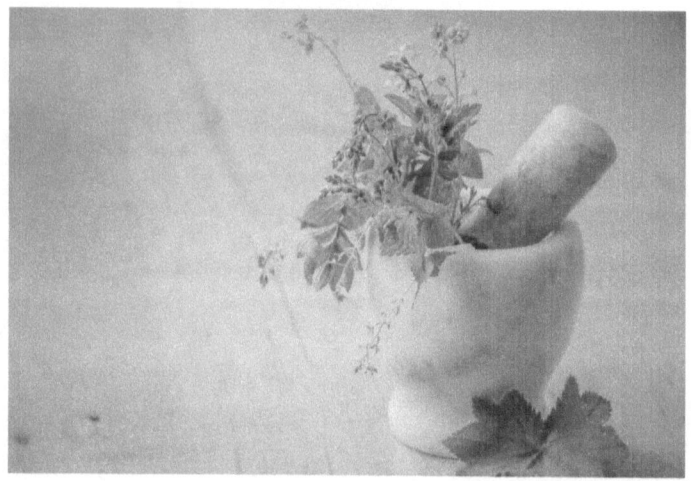

Before you start a remedy, ensure you have everything you need – the ingredients, the tools, and the storage containers.

You want to follow a recipe from start to finish with no interruption.

Never take shortcuts and never substitute ingredients. Also, be precise when you measure those ingredients.

Always get the right containers. In some cases, dark glass bottles are required, and you can get these online or at most health food stores.

Read the instructions through before you start a

recipe and look up anything that you don't understand.

Don't rush; herbal medicine takes time to get right, and each step is precise.

Be positive and remove all potential distractions. You must be focused only on the task at hand.

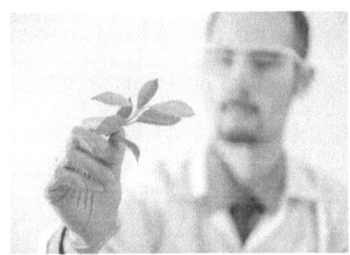

You could also consider taking an in depth video course on herbal medicines to expand your knowledge beyond what you learn in this guide.

Amazing herbal courses can be found online, as well as webinars and even DVDs. Some are free, and most are inexpensive.

Make remedies in advance of when you need them. For example, flu remedies should be made before flu season starts; that way, when your symptoms start, you can take your remedy straight away.

Make teas, tinctures, and ointments in advance,

so you don't need to go shopping or make them when you are not feeling well.

Label your remedies with the name, the date you made it, and the expiry date if there is one.

Set aside an area to store your remedies and keep them separate from everything else.

Your kitchen must be spotless, as must your prep area and the tools you use. Make sure you wash your hands before you start and after you finish. Before you start making a remedy, sterilize your tools and storage containers.

Either immerse them in a bowl of boiling water for five minutes and then lay them on clean towels to dry, or use the dishwasher to wash everything and then pour boiling water over the top before you use them.

These are just a few important tips when it comes to making herbal medicines.

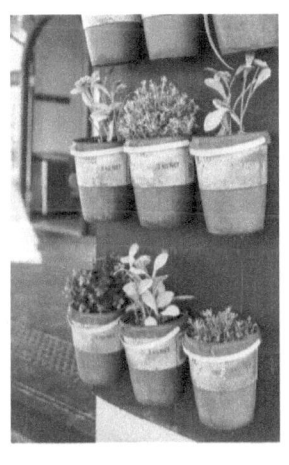

Growing herbs is very simple, so long as you know how to do it and your herbal starter plants are provided with the right growing conditions.

If you do decide to make an herb garden you'll also get the added benefit of having organic, home-grown herbs that you can use in your cooking too.

Be aware that not all herbs grow in all conditions, and some will be better grown indoors.

Doing this saves you a lot of money on buying

the remedies, and this is really only the start. Herbs also repel pests and attract beneficial insects. Plus, any gardening, even if it is just in containers, is good for the mind, body, and soul.

If certain herbs just do not grow in your area, you may be just as well to purchase them as and when you need them. Most herbal remedies can be made with dried herbs, and these do store well.

Be aware that herbs require care, especially if they are grown in containers or indoors.

This is a problem if you are constantly traveling, so try to find someone who can care for them when you are not there.

However, no matter how much effort you put in, some herbs will fail; don't be discouraged, just try again.

It can also be tough work to put in an herb garden, especially if the ground needs clearing first. Get some help and stick at it; it will be worth it in the end.

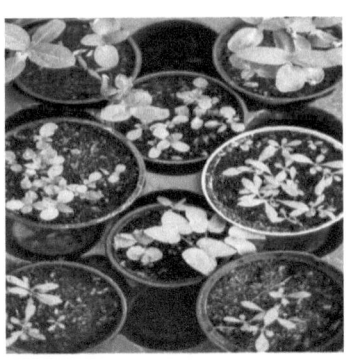

Tips on Growing an Herb Garden

If you have never done any gardening, read some books or research on the Internet first. Get it the right first time, and you won't have to redo your work.

An herb garden isn't just useful; it should look appealing to look at and easy to work.

Read up on plants that need full sun, those that will do well in shade or partial shade, learn about companion planting and plan your garden well.

Plant according to your planting zone – you can find out what this is on the internet. That way, you will only plant herbs that have the best chance of success. If you buy plants, make sure they are organic and look healthy.

Be sure to read up on how far apart to plant your

herbs and how deep. If you are starting from seed, its best to start in pots; that way, you can thin out the seedlings and ensure you bring on only the strongest of plants.

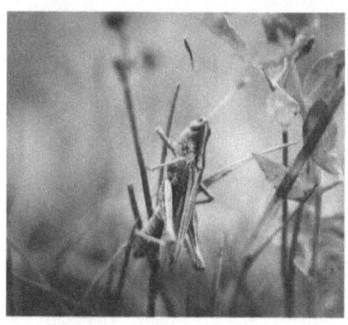

Learn how to protect your plants from disease and pests – companion planting will help you here.

If you are planting in containers, make sure they are cleaned and sterilized first, to eliminate the risk of contamination or disease from old soil.

Protect plants from frost, especially young ones. You can purchase garden fleece quite cheaply on the Internet or use row covers or small clay pots.

Always mark the plants, so you know what they are.

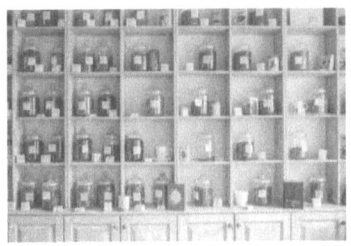

Create your own compost heap, so you have healthy compost to feed your plants with.

Some herbs, particularly mint, are invasive; if you don't want them taking over your garden, plant them in containers.

If you are going to dry the herbs, you harvest, make an area that is warm and well-ventilated where the herbs can be hung for drying.

Basic Tools for Creating Herbal Remedies

Making herbal remedies requires some basic tools, including measuring and weighing devices, tools for chopping and cutting, and more.

You may already have these tools in your kitchen but, if you are going to get serious about making your own herbal medicines, you might want to consider, eventually, buying equipment that you only use for that, keeping it separate from your kitchen.

You should also ensure that you have a supply of basic pantry items – good-quality vodka, beeswax, organic honey, coconut oil, white vinegar, and good quality olive oil for starters.

Make sure your tools are sterilized before you use them and never reuse fabrics, such as towels, without washing and sterilizing them first.

If you use cheesecloth, never reuse it; together with the herbs you strain out, it can go in your compost bin.

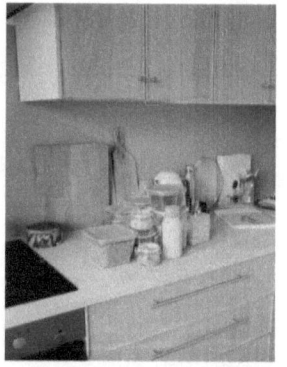

Essential Tools for Herbal Remedies:

- **Blender/Food Processor** – useful when you have a lot of herbs to chop.
- **Capsules** – you can buy these online in different sizes and quantities. They are ideal for encapsulating powdered herbs

(you will want a small funnel or an encapsulation tool which you can buy with the capsules).

- **Cheesecloth** – essential for poultices and useful for straining herbs. Buy it in bulk online and keep it sealed in a container, so it doesn't get dusty or dirty.
- **Cutting Boards** – do not use these for any purpose other than with your herbal remedies otherwise you run the risk of cross-contamination.
- **Sieve** – as fine a mesh as you can get, so you can separate herbs and liquid quickly. You can buy them in all different sizes so get whatever sizes you need.
- **Funnels** – try to get stainless-steel or glass funnels in different sizes.
- **Glass Containers** – preferably with tight lids. These are used to store dried herbs or for when a recipe, such as a tincture, needs to be left for a while. Enclose each container in a dark sock to keep the light out. You can also use dark glass bottles with tight lids to store your made remedies in. Again, these can all be purchased online

- **Heavy-duty Stainless-Steel Pans –** your pans must be nonreactive and heavy-duty, especially as some concoctions require boiling for some time. You can also use ceramic-coated or cast-iron. DO NOT use Teflon, aluminum, or copper. You should also consider putting some tools aside for use purely when you use heavy oils and waxes; never use these for cooking or for water-based remedies afterward.
- **Labels –** you should always label your medicines, so you know what they are, when you made them and when they expire.
- **Mixing Bowls –** again, use stainless-steel or glass and get some different sizes. Plastic is not recommended as it can leach toxins into your medicines.
- **Scraping and Mixing Tools –** silicone spatulas and stainless-steel whisks are best for mixing and scraping the sides of your pans and bowls. Get them in multiple sizes to make sure you have what you need.

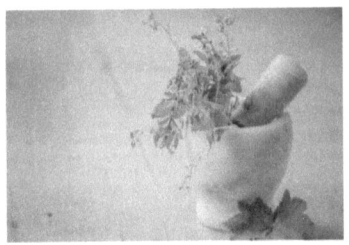

- **Salve Tins/Balm Jars** – you can get these online and are ideal for small amounts of balm and ointments.
- **Kitchen Scale** – this must be accurate, have ounces as a measurement, and be food safe.
- **Knives** – sharp ones so you can easily chop fresh herbs. Get ones with a non-serrated blade and heavy handles and get a knife sharpener so you can keep them sharp.
- **Tea Infuser** – makes it easier for preparing loose-leaf tea.

Internal and External Medicines

Internal medicines are typically swallowed, such as lozenges, tinctures, and teas, or inhaled, usually via hot steam. External herbal medicines are applied to your skin, usually for minor injuries, skin complaints or sore muscles, itching and burning, such as herbal baths, salves, and ointments.

Herbal Baths

Warm water is great for cleansing the body, soothing aching muscles, and relaxing your mind, and adding herbs can even help you address health concerns.

You can use fresh herbs or dried, essential oils, Dead Sea salts, Epsom salts, and so on in your bath.

Always stay in an herbal bath for at least 15 minutes; you can add more hot water if needed. Don't take hot baths too often as they dry your skin out and make sure you apply a good moisturizer afterward.

Tips for Herbal Baths

- Start running your bath and add about ½ a cup of dried or fresh herbs while the tap is running.
- To make them easier to clean up, wrap them in cheesecloth and tie them under the water stream. Then allow them the bag to float in the bath and discard it when you have finished.
- Prepare a decoction by placing ½ cup of dried or fresh herbs in a pot with 2 or 3 cups of cold water. Bring to a boil and then reduce the heat; cover and simmer for about 15 to 20 minutes. Pour it into your bath through a fine sieve.
- Make an infusion by putting about ½ a cup of dried or fresh herbs in a stainless-

steel bowl and adding 3 cups of boiling water. Cover and leave to infuse for about 15 or 20 minutes, then pour into the bath through a fine sieve.

Pills and Capsules

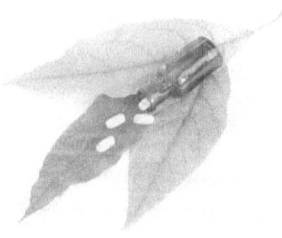

Pills are more difficult to make than capsules, and they take longer, but you don't need to purchase empty capsules to fill. Both are cheap to make and easy to swallow.

Before you make pills or capsules, ensure the dosage is correct. Each pill or capsule must contain the entire dose or a standard portion of a dose – a half or a quarter of a dose, for example.

Make sure you label the container they are being stored in and include the dosage per pill or capsule. And, if there are any contraindications or cautionary instructions, add those too.

Tips for Capsules

- Purchase empty capsules – you can get these online, along with a capsule filling tool. This will make the job quicker and easier.
- If you don't get the filler tool, you will need to use the two halves of the capsule to scoop up your powder before pushing the ends together – this is not a precise method, and you may also crush the capsules.
- If you do not have ready-powdered herbs to put in the capsules, you will need to grind your herbs first – a coffee grinder or pestle and mortar will do the trick.
- You can choose between gelatin (animal matter) and cellulose (vegetarian) capsules – try to get the vegetarian ones as they are natural and have no preservatives.
- A 00-size capsule should hold 500 mg of powdered herbs, and they are the easiest to fill. If you struggle with large capsules, go for a 0-size, half the size of the 00-size.

Tips for Pills

- Use fine-ground herbs as the resulting pill is less likely to crumble than if you use coarse-ground herbs.
- ¼ cup of inert powder, such as stevia, acacia, slippery elm or arrowroot, should be used with each ¾ cup of ground active herbs to help bind the herbs together.
- You need good math skills to work out how much mixture goes into each pill; this will depend on the active herb's dosage. Keep in mind that the ratio is 1-part inactive herb to 3-parts active.
- Use small batches, so the mixture doesn't dry too quickly. Form the pills by rolling the mixture into a ball and flattening it slightly. Lay them on parchment paper and bake at around 200°F – the pills need to dry completely, so bake for about 10 minutes and check them. Repeat until you are happy.
- Always label your pill bottles with dosage and cautions.
- Use glass bottles with airtight lids and store in a cool dark place.
- If you need to use fresh herbs, only make

enough pills to last a few days – the fresh herbs break down much quicker.

Decoctions and Confusions

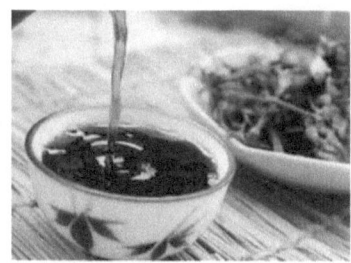

Both of these are similar to herbal teas, prepared with boiling water, and can be made using dried or fresh herbs. They are a great way of getting fast relief for sore throats, congestion, indigestion, and other common ailments.

Decoctions and infusion differ in the plant parts used. Decoctions are made from roots, bark, and stems, although you can add leaves if they are tough or thick. Infusions are normally made from the above-ground parts, such as buds, flowers, light leaves, and stems.

You can also chill a decoction or infusion and use it for treating burns, rashes, minor cuts, bug bites, headaches, and mild skin infections.

Tips for Making Decoctions and Confusions

- For infusions, chop or crush the herbs and place them in a diffuser inside a mug or bowl. Add a cup of boiling water and cover; leave to steep for 15 to 20 minutes before using.
- For decoctions, chop fresh roots or parts finely; if using dried plant parts, grind or crush them. Add the amount needed to a pan with a cup of cold water and gradually heat the water to a boil. Cover, reduce heat and leave to simmer for about 15 to 20 minutes.
- Use filtered water for decoctions and infusions.
- Both will last in the refrigerator for up to five days, stored in sealed containers.
- For topical use, decant the infusion or decoction to a clean, new spray bottle or a glass bottle and use a cotton ball or soft cloth to apply it. The spray bottle method is best for large areas of burned or irritated skin

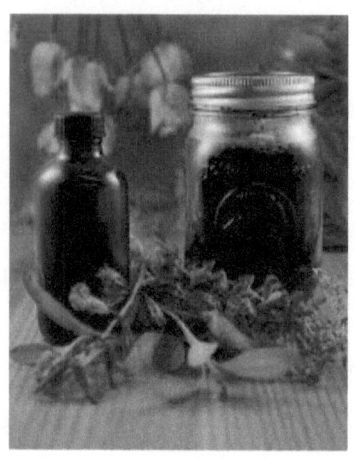

Liniments

Herbal liniments are good for sprains, bruises, sore muscles, and joints. Usually, an apple cider vinegar base is used, or a base of oil or vodka.

The herbs are either intensely warming or cooling, such as cayenne, peppermint, or ginger. Prepared liniments should be stored in a cool dark place and can be kept for up to 2 years. They take a while to make, so prepare them in advance of when you are likely to need them.

Tips for Making Liniments

- Choose your recipe and sterilize your equipment, including a dark glass jar. Put the herbs in the jar, add the base, and seal the jar. Store it in a dark, room-temperature place.
- It should be left for around 8 weeks to cure but, if desperate, you can use it after about 10 days. Once a day, give the jar a vigorous shake.
- When it has cured, strain it through multiple cheesecloth layers and squeeze as much liquid as you can out. Decant to a dark jar, label it and store it.

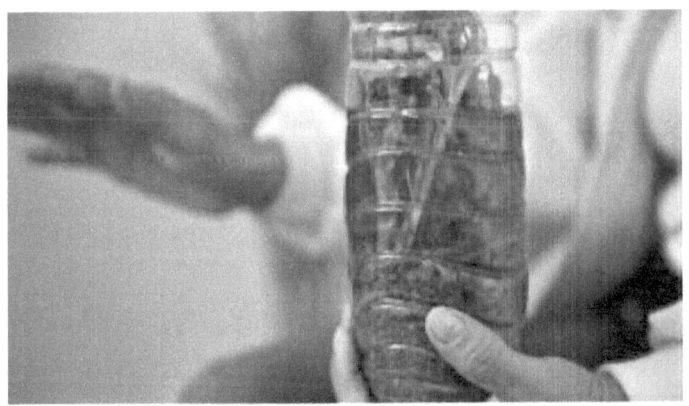

If this is your first time using a new recipe, test it on the inside bend of your elbow. Leave it for 12

hours or more; if a rash appears, scrub the area with soap and water and throw the liniment out.

If you want a more intense effect from a liniment, apply it to the area and cover it with a thick piece of cloth; this stops it from evaporating so quickly.

Always use dried herbs; fresh herbs spoil while the liniment is curing.

And lastly, don't apply a liniment to sensitive skin and keep it away from your eyes and nose. If the liniment is for dry skin, use vinegar or oil as your base.

Lozenges

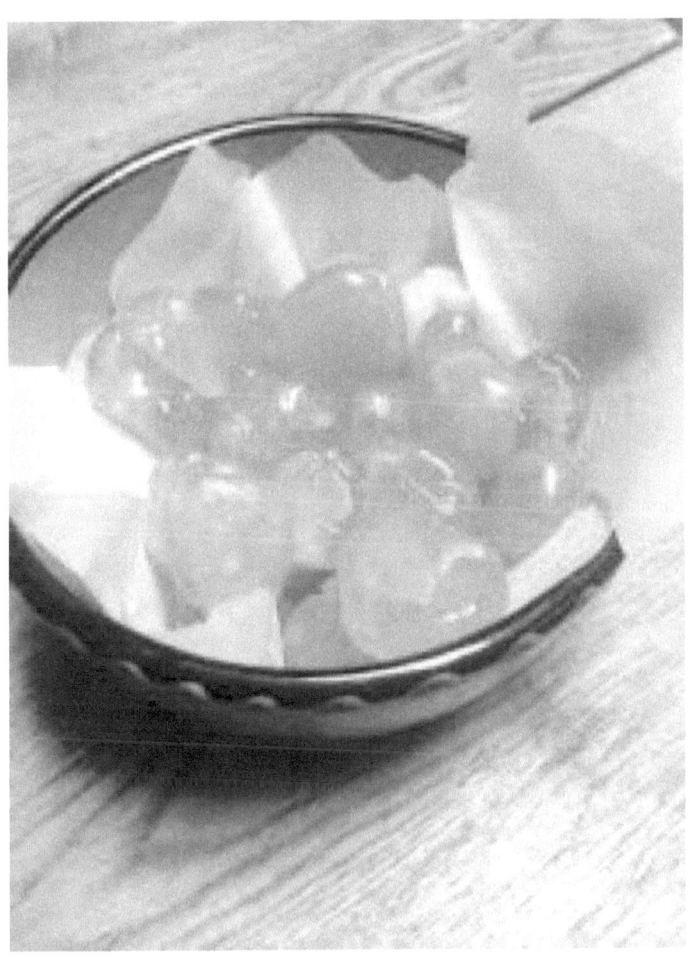

Lozenges are much like cough drops or hard candy but, rather than chemicals and preservatives, they have healing herbs in them.

Lozenge Tips and Tricks

- If you already make candy, these should be a piece of cake. If not, be prepared for some difficulty. If you make mistakes, don't be hard on yourself. Try to focus on the thermometer, keep the heat right, and you'll soon get it.
- You need about an hour of uninterrupted time – the herbal infusion will take about 20 minutes and another half hour to get to the right temperature. Once you pour it, the lozenges won't take long to set.
- When they are set, toss them in powdered stevia to stop them from sticking together.
- They should cure for an hour or more at room temperature before you store them. This stops heat escaping and stops a build-up of condensation. If you do get condensation, the lozenges will stick together.
- You can store them in tightly sealed jars or tins in the freezer or refrigerator.
- Do be careful not to burn yourself when making lozenges. If you do spill boiling liquid on your skin, immediately run cold water over it and remove the substance

from your skin. If you don't act quickly enough, you can be burned seriously.

To make lozenges, you will need a candy thermometer that has a clip on it, so you can attach it to your pan, a baking sheet that has raised edges, a silicone baking mat, or parchment paper, or you can use small silicone candy molds.

Powders

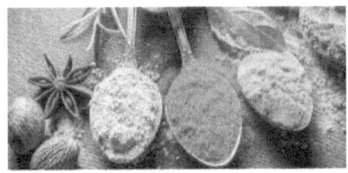

Herbal powders work well for ringworm, athlete's foot, and other skin ailments. You can also use them to absorb sweat and ensure body odor is kept under control, great to use during the summer months.

Nice-smelling body powders can be made using baking soda or arrowroot powder with fine white clay, or you can grind herbs into a very fine powder and apply them directly to the area you want.

Tips for Powders

- Start by choosing your recipe and grind the required herbs to a fine powder. Combine the powder with the other ingredients carefully.
- Transfer the herbs to a container using a funnel. One of the best containers is a sugar or saltshaker.
- When you want to use it, just shake it onto the affected area, just as you would talcum powder.

Some of the best herbs to use are peppermint, lavender, and rose petals. And if you add a few drops of a matching essential oil, you can boost the scent and take advantage of a bit of aromatherapy at the same time.

Herbal powders do not remain efficient for long, and this is down to the herbs being ground. Only make what you can use in a few days and then make another batch when you need it. If you make an aromatic powder, the smell will last longer, so long as it is stored in a sealed container in a cool dark place.

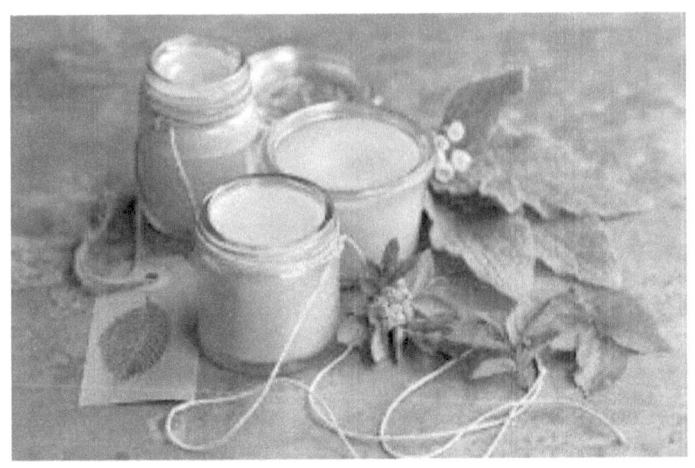

Salves and Ointments

Both of these are viscous preparations with an oil base, and you can use just about medicinal herb you like, so long as it is suitable for topical use. Both sales and ointments are good for dry skin, minor cuts, scrapes, chapped areas, and sunburned areas.

Tips for Salves and Ointments

- It doesn't matter what herbs you choose to use in an ointment or salve; the basic preparation is the same, ensuring that you retain as high a level of the healing compounds as possible and make it the consistency you want.

- Start by adding 4 cups of fresh herbs OR 1 cup of dried herbs to 4 cups of water. Gradually bring it to a boil, reduce the heat and simmer until the liquid has reduced by around 50%. There is no need to cover the pan. Turn the heat off and leave it to cool.
- When it has cooled, you can strain the liquid through multiple layers of cheesecloth into a stainless-steel or glass bowl. Squeeze the cloth to get as much liquid out of the herbs as you can and then discard the cloth and herbs, either in the bin or into your compost heap. If you opt to use a nut milk bag, you can wash it and reuse it for another preparation at a later time.
- Next, decant the liquid into a measuring cup, noting the amount you have. Pour into a heavy pan you use for heating waxes and oils. If this is your first time working with those, choose a pan that you can reserve just for use with the wax and oil – no matter how much you scrub it, you will

still get an oily layer, and you don't want that contaminating a non-oil-based herbal mixture.

- Pour out the oil you are using to the same measure as the liquid. Use sunflower, olive, sweet almond, or jojoba oil. Add it to the pan, stir and bring to a simmer. Leave it, so the water evaporates, stirring it on occasion.

- Once the water is gone, add pure beeswax – just enough to get it to the consistency you want. Stir it thoroughly, ensuring everything is mixed together and then decant into glass containers. Leave it to cool completely before capping the containers with tight-fitting lids. Label them and store them somewhere dark and cool.

PART II
COMMON MEDICINAL HERBS

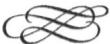

A medicinal plant is any plant which, in one or more of its organs, contains substances that can be used for therapeutic purposes or which are precursors for the synthesis of useful drugs.

This description makes it possible to distinguish between medicinal plants whose therapeutic properties and constituents have been established scientifically, and plants that are regarded as medicinal but which have not yet been subjected to a thorough scientific study.

Here are a few interesting statistics about the global herb market, these statistics are made primarily from the common medicinal herbs I will discuss in this chapter.

The growing importance of medicinal plants can be appreciated from the economic stand point when the following facts are considered:

- Global trade in herbs is over USD 100 Billion per annum
- India and China's medicinal plant trade is about two to five billion US dollars annually
- In Germany, it is over one billion US dollars annually
- Rose Periwinkle which is endemic to Madagascar fetches US $100 million per annum
- China trades in 7,000 species and 700,000 tons of medicinal plants per annum
- India trades in 7,000 species of medicinal plants
- Morocco exports 58.7 tons of medicinal plants annually
- In the last 5 years, sales of medicinal plants doubled in China, tripled in India and grew by 25% in Europe.

In this section we will look at the most common medicinal herbs and cover a lot of questions that may have been unanswered up until now. Questions such as, what are the most common medicinal herbs? Where can I find them? Is it better to grow them or buy them?

So many people who want to get into herbal medicine and don't have the faintest clue in where to start.

One of the best long term strategy is to take a chance and start your very own herb garden. What we need to do ultimately is to secure a magnificent supply.

The best way to do that is to grow your own herbs; even if you don't have an aptitude for plants, the best time to start learning is now. You may even find you have an affinity for growing herbs!

After you get your various medicinal herbs settled in, most of your herbs will grow with little or no help from you. Just don't forget to give them some love sometimes and the occasional watering.

The trouble is, there are so many useful herbs, it's hard to know where to start. Because this topic can be so overwhelming and many people would like a short and effective plan to follow, I picked just 20 of the most popular herbs to get you started:

How did I narrow the list down to 20? This guide focuses on the twenty herbs described below based on the following criteria:

- The herbs selected are the easiest to grow.
- The herbs selected are the easiest to forage.
- The herbs selected have great qualities.
- The herbs selected can be useful for a huge number of medicinal herbal remedies.

On that last point, if you grow an herb that only has one real use, you have to seriously think about whether it is worth the effort to plant and harvest it or whether it would just be easier to buy it when you need it.

All the herbs I list below are medicinal in nature, and most can be grown just about anywhere. If you can't grow them, you should be able to buy them easily enough. So, lets walk through these amazing herbs that will change your life forever!

The 20 Best Medicinal Herbs to Get Started

. . .

Calendula

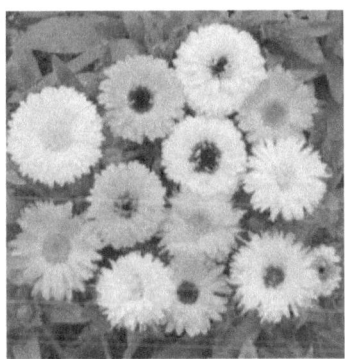

Calendula is a fantastic herb to grow, a beautiful yellow or orange flower that is packed with medicinal qualities. It grows like mad and will grow anywhere; as a bonus, it's one of the top plants for bringing in the bees.

Calendula has many properties, including healing and strengthening for the skin. The easiest thing in the world is to pick the flowers and leave them infusing in olive oil for when you are ready to use it in soaps, salves, and other useful products.

Another bonus with calendula is that the flower is edible and will soon brighten up any salad.

. . .

Cayenne

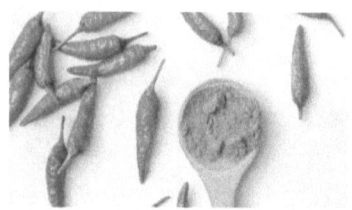

Cayenne is another herb that is dead simple to grow and should be a part of every garden. For those that don't know, cayenne is a hot red pepper, a very pretty plant, and is great for adding spice to any dish. And, once established, it will grow like mad, especially if you live in a warm climate, and the peppers are easy to dry.

In terms of healing properties, cayenne is excellent for boosting circulation, can help slow a heart attack while you wait for help, and, as a hemostatic herb, it can also help stop bleeding.

Chamomile

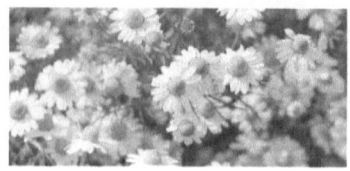

No herb garden would be complete without chamomile, and most of you have heard of it for two reasons – chamomile lawns and chamomile tea, the latter of which is a great de-stressing and calming drink. The chamomile flowers have a scent of honey and taste sweet.

As well as being a mild sedative and relaxant, chamomile is also an excellent anti-inflammatory, containing high azulene levels. It can help relieve pain, especially in arthritis, and is a great drink before you go to bed as it can help you to sleep better.

Chamomile isn't easy to grow if you live in a hot climate; although it loves being in full sun, it isn't fond of heat.

However, given the right climate, chamomile is simple to grow because you can grow it in bad soil, and you don't need to provide fertilization.

Chickweed

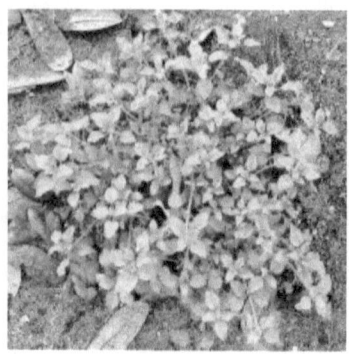

Chickweed is one of the most misunderstood herbs of all time, but it has some great medicinal properties.

The Latin name for chickweed is Stellaria, which means star, and it was named for its beautiful white flowers that look like little stars. It is one of the easiest of herbs to grow and has plenty of uses.

Chickweed is high in nutrition and is a diuretic, making it an excellent choice for kidney and liver health. And it works well in salves used for healing eczema, dry skin, rashes, and other skin complaints.

Dandelion

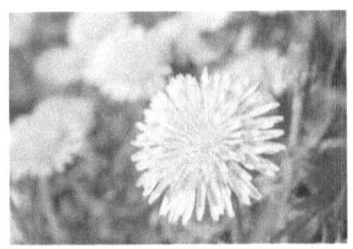

Dandelion is considered by many people as a weed, but it is one of the oldest and most powerful of all the medicinal herbs. It's another herb with diuretic properties, making it great for kidney and liver health.

You can eat dandelion too. The roots can be roasted and added to tea and coffee, and you can add the leaves to your salads and other foods too. Dandelion grows everywhere, even where you don't want them too, so if you don't have any growing in your yard, just head out along the country paths and roadsides – you'll find plenty there.

Feverfew

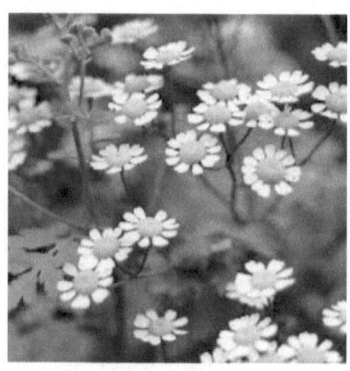

Feverfew is a beautiful plant with white flowers, but, in some climates, it can be rather invasive; give it half a chance, and it will take over your yard.

However, it does have many medicinal uses. Firstly, the name gives away that it works well to reduce a fever.

But now it has become popular as an aid to preventing migraines and reducing the time and intensity of them when you do get them.

One of the best ways to do this is to make a tea with 1-part feverfew, 1-part lemon balm, and 1-part spearmint. It is a calming, nervine tea that you can drink every day. Feverfew can also be made into a tincture for bug bites and has mild properties for relieving pain.

Feverfew has lovely white flowers, and at least where I live, is rather invasive. I don't mind, though,

. . .

Garlic

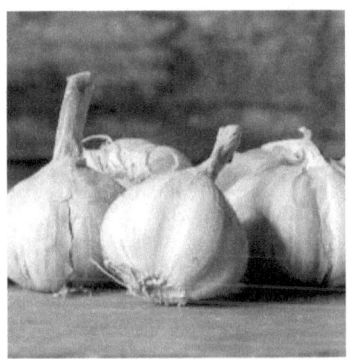

Garlic should be grown in every garden, given that it is one of the best herbs to grow and is a good all-rounder. You can use garlic to treat flu, colds, a sore throat, even digestive problems. And because garlic can help stimulate white blood cells, it is a great immune system booster.

It doesn't stop there. As well as being incredibly flavorful in many dishes, it also has antibacterial, antiseptic, and vermifuge properties and can be used as a blood purifier and to help with blood circulation. Lastly, if you have type 2 diabetes, garlic can help keep your blood sugar levels regulated.

. . .

Ginger

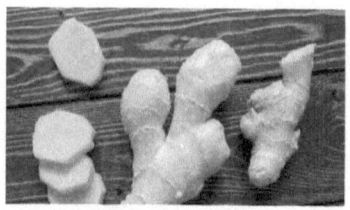

Ginger is another herb that everyone should have in their yard. It isn't a root, even though it is known as gingerroot; it is a rhizome. The confusion comes from the fact that the useful part of the plant is grown underground.

Ginger is a stimulant and goes great in teas, fermented foods, and tinctures, as well as being used in cooking.

It has anti-inflammatory, decongestant properties and is great for creating warmth and boosting circulation. It's also good for stomach issues, including flatulence and nausea.

If you live in a cool climate, you will need to grow ginger indoors or in a greenhouse as it loves a hot, humid, tropical environment.

Lavender

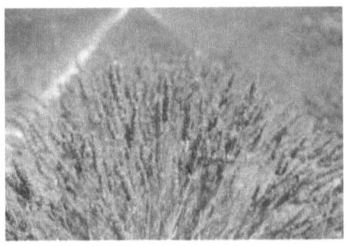

Lavender has so many uses; not only does it smell gorgeous; it attracts bees, and it has some great medicinal uses.

It's also used as an air freshener and a way of cleaning the air in small, enclosed spaces, like drawers. It doesn't like a harsh winter or cold wind, so you may need to invest in garden fleece to protect your plants.

Lavender is typically used as a calming agent and goes well in teas and bath products, as well as hand and skin salves.

Lemon Balm

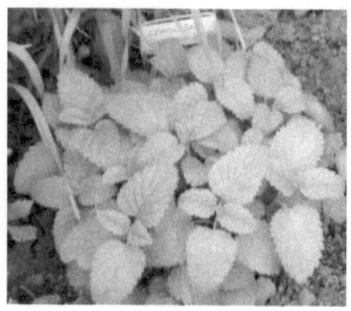

Lemon balm is part of the mint family, and true to the family, it spreads like wildfire.

This is another herb that the bees love, it smells gorgeous, and it grows almost anywhere. Another thing that makes it so great is the feeling you get when working with it.

It tastes lemony and is an excellent addition to herb teas, not just in nutritional terms, but the relaxing, calming properties it offers too.

Marshmallow

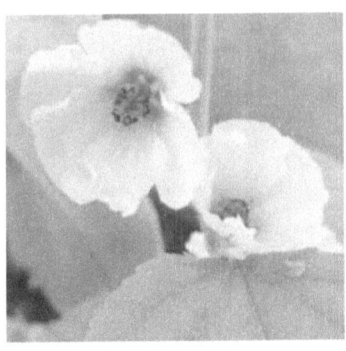

Not many people grow this, but it is a very popular herb. As well as providing the perfect complement to hot herbs, it is soothing and a demulcent, which means it has anti-inflammatory properties.

It is particularly soothing for inflammation inside the mucous membranes and is a great herb to add to herbal teas and blends specifically for inflammation.

You can also dry the root and make it into a paste to treat burns.

Marshmallow looks very much like a smaller version of hollyhock, and, in actual fact, if you grow hollyhocks, you can use those instead of marshmallow, as they have a similar chemical constituency.

The whole marshmallow plant is edible, and you can add the flowers to your salads.

· · ·

Mullein

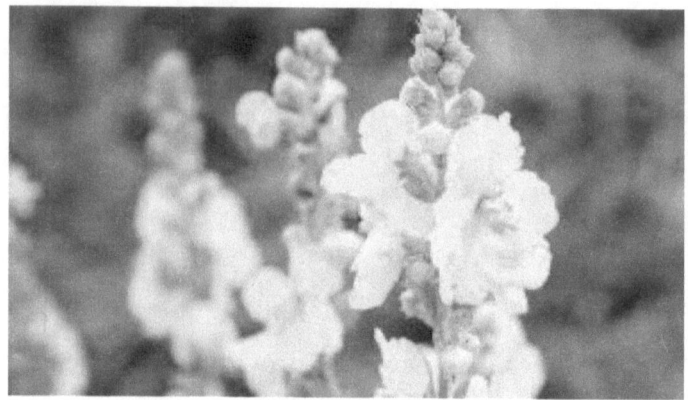

Mullein is also commonly seen as a weed but is another wonderful medicinal herb. It certainly wouldn't be considered your average dig up and throw away weed that constantly plagues your lawn.

It grows into a tall stem, sometimes up to 7-feet tall with pretty yellow flowers—it like full sun, plenty of water, and not too hot a climate.

Mullein is a great herb for people with respiratory illnesses, including lung, breathing, and sinus problems.

It can be used as a tincture or made into a tea, and the large leaves do well as a poultice covering in an emergency.

. . .

Oregano

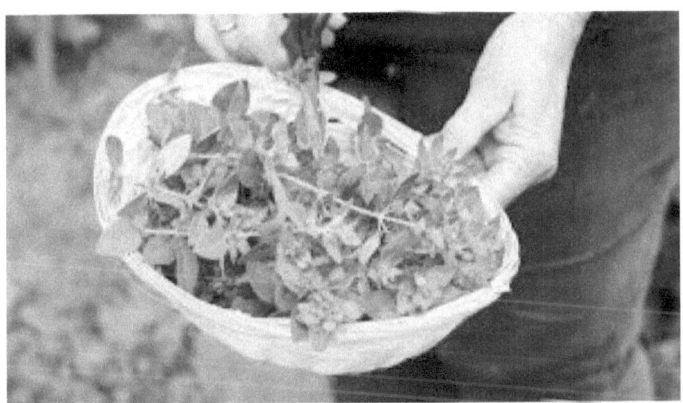

Oregano is one of those herbs that, when it gets going, there's no stopping it – unless you know how to.

It is fantastic to use in cooking and works well on Mediterranean foods.

It likes a warm, dry climate, but is hardy and can survive a winter that doesn't drop below freezing.

As a medicinal herb, oregano has antibiotic, antiviral, and antifungal properties and has a high level of antioxidants.

It's also a great herb for skincare and for healing digestive issues.

. . .

Peppermint

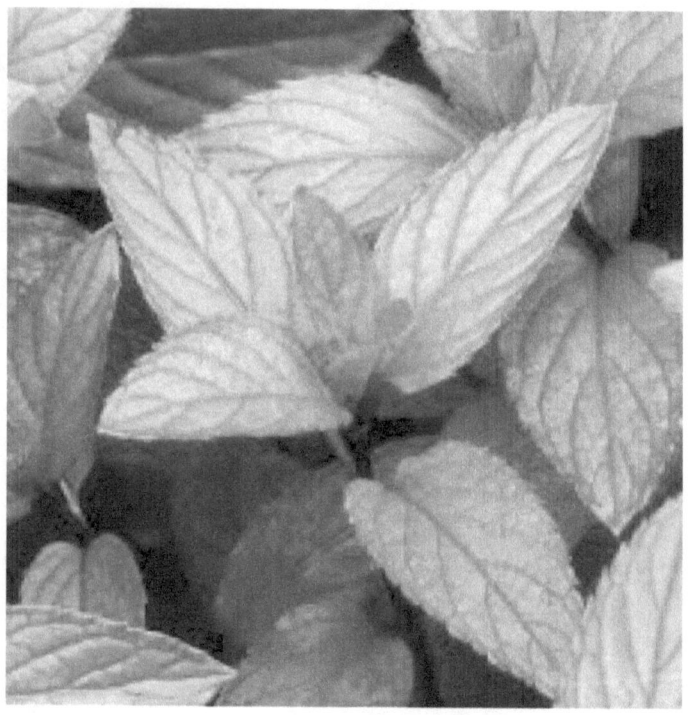

Mint grows everywhere and anywhere, and it spreads like wildfire. Leave it planted in the garden, and it will take over.

If you're happy with that, fine; if not, plant it in pots. In medicinal terms, peppermint is a great digestive aid and helps to get rid of flatulence.

It is also mildly anti-spasmodic, so it is useful for menstrual, digestive, and other types of cramps.

Plantain

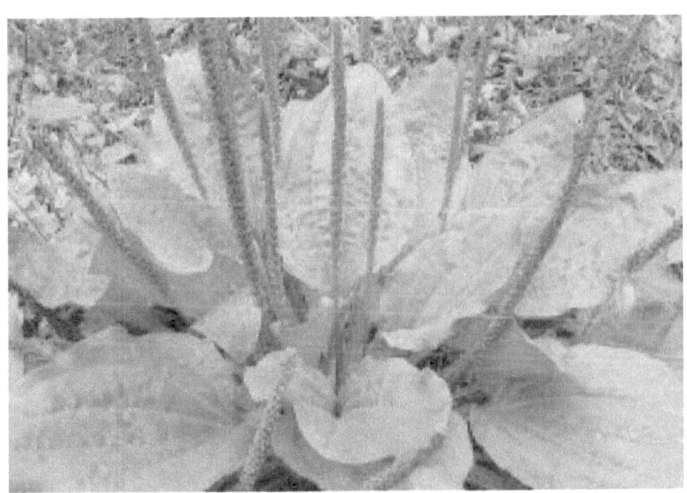

Plantain is another herb that many people turn their nose up, seeing it as nothing more than a weed when it is actually very useful.

Plantain is one of those herbs that grow all over the place and is a job to get rid of once it is settled in your garden.

It is good for liver health, blood cleansing, and detoxification and can be infused easily in oil to make it into a healing salve. Plantain is also an edible herb.

. . .

Rosemary

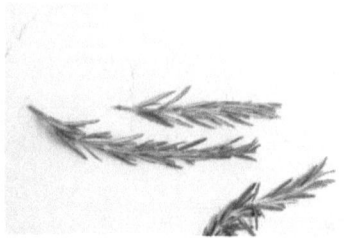

Everyone has heard of rosemary, and many of us have used it in our cooking. But rosemary is more than just a culinary herb; it is also well known for its ability to help improve memory function.

It is an antioxidant with mildly analgesic properties, which means it offers pain relief.

It also helps raise blood pressure and boost circulation and is commonly known as a stimulant herb.

Anyone with high blood pressure should take care when using rosemary for medicinal purposes.

Rosemary likes the climate hot and dry, but you can get it through the winter if you bring it indoors or wrap it in garden fleece throughout the colder months.

St. John's Wort

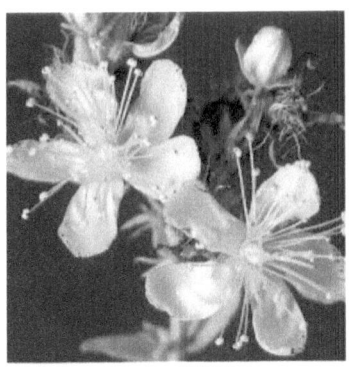

This is one of the more misunderstood plants. A few years back, it was popular and was being shouted from the rooftops as a natural anti-depressant. However, while it can provide some relief for sadness, mild depression, grief, and SAD (Seasonal Affective Disorder), it certainly is not a full-on anti-depressant.

One thing you do need to know about this herb is that it interacts with certain drugs, so do NOT use it without speaking to your doctor first. To be honest, you should do that as a matter of course, before using any herb for medicinal purposes.

St. John's Wort does work for neuralgia and helps to relieve both sciatica and back pain. It prefers a cooler, temperate climate and is a pretty plant for any garden. It works well as an herb-infused oil, which can be used as a base for salves and ointments.

Another word of warning; it does have photo-toxic properties and can harm any animals that graze on it too much.

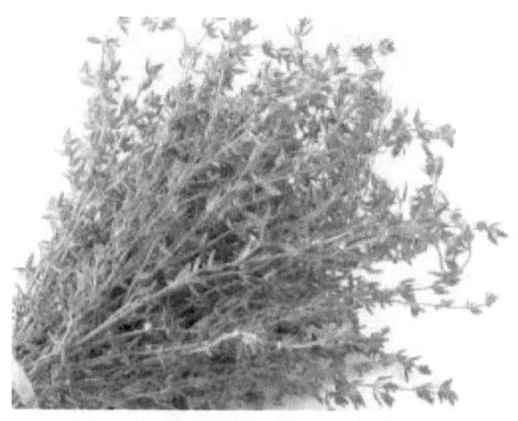

Thyme

Thyme is an excellent herb for any garden; it smells gorgeous, attracts the bees, and can easily be used in cooking as well as for medicinal purposes.

A small plant, thyme spreads quite quickly and is pretty hardy.

It works well to ease the symptoms of flu and colds and can also be used to ward off a cold int eh first place.

Thyme has disinfectant properties and works

well as a mouth gargle for sore throats and as a skin wash for infections.

There are many different types of thyme, but the best ones for the medicinal herb garden are Thymus citriodorus and Thymus vulgaris.

Valerian

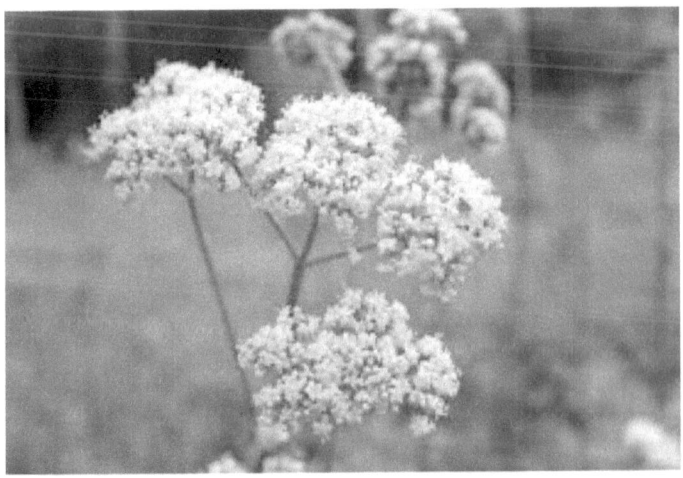

Valerian is a stately plant that can grow to heights of 4-feet tall with clusters of white lacy flowers. It is a strong sedative but safe to use and can help relieve pain, insomnia, and feelings of anxiety and stress.

However, it doesn't work for everyone and can

have the opposite effect. If you are trying it out, do so on an evening when you don't need to be anywhere the following day.

Yarrow

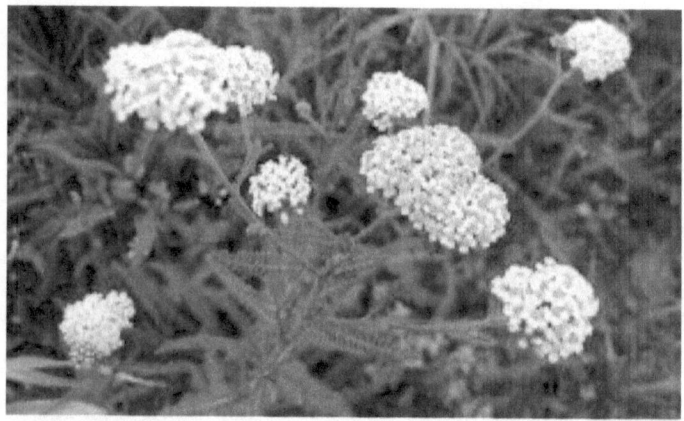

Yarrow used to be called the Battlefield flower, especially during the Civil War, and it can help to heal injuries and clot wounds.

It is a hemostatic herb and can also help to reduce fever, fight off colds, and relieve the symptoms of hay fever.

However, it can induce sweating, so if you are already suffering from a hot fever, it probably isn't the best to use.

It is a nice plant to grow, with grey, feathery leaves, and bunches of small flowers.

At this point I've covered the 20 medicinal herbs that we will be working with and we should be ready to move on!

Final Thoughts on This 20 Herb Selection

There are literally hundreds of medicinal herbs. In a beginner's guide there is simply no place for making an attempt at going over all of them as you'll see in the recipe section these herbs can do remarkable healing when used in the proper manner.

That being said, it is still a great idea to do thorough research before planting an herb garden.

There may be herbs that I haven't listed here which could particularly suit the environment you live in or the types of ailments common in your region.

I encourage you when selecting herbs to really think hard about what you will need them for.

Create a shortlist of plants and look at your planting zone to see what will and won't grow.

In some cases, you may need to invest in a greenhouse. In almost every case, you will simply need to experiment with what works and what doesn't.

It is my hope that you really learned a lot in this section and now have a good idea of what some of the very best medicinal herbs truly are, what they look like and where you can usually find them.

Take a trip to your grocery store, your local nursery and your local farmer's market, make a list of what is available and try to get your head around where you can get these herbs and the seeds or starter plants to grow these herbs yourself.

PART III
HERBAL REMEDIES FOR
COMMON AILMENTS

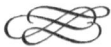

When it comes to creating herbal remedies, a lot of it amounts to trial and error. Just like riding a bike, it takes practice to get an amazing result or consistent results each time.

You undoubtedly will need to determine the best method based on the herb itself, and the condition you are treating. Be especially careful when you're cooking herbs.

If you get above the degradation point of the essential oils within the herbs, then the oils may lose potency.

Preparing medicinal herbs is a skill that should be practiced on a regular basis. Add to your knowledge through research of herbal medicine guides and recipes, as well as experimentation.

Now it's time to whip up an herbal remedy!

The recipes I've selected to share with you here are simple to make while at the same time very effective and soothing.

Read the instructions, get your ingredients together, and remember that making your own natural herbal remedies and medicines should be fun!

Deep Detox and Soothing Ginger Infusion

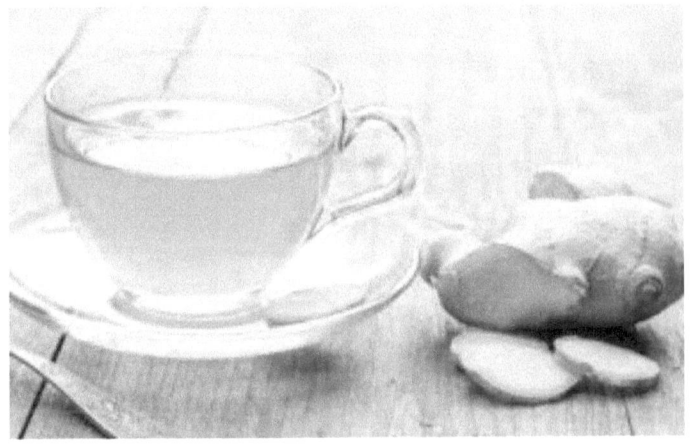

The history of Ginger (Zingiber officinalis) began

5,000 years ago, when Indians and ancient Chinese considered it a root tonic and good for many diseases.

The ginger is originally from Southeast Asia but has long been cultivated in other countries.

Ginger tea is fantastic for nausea, heartburn, and acid reflux, as well as being effective against morning sickness. If you have a tummy ache or any of the symptoms mentioned above

Ingredients:

- 8 oz. water
- 2-inch piece of ginger root
- Honey or stevia to provide sweetness – optional

Instructions:

1. Put the water onto boil and peel your gingerroot. Slice it very thin and place in a teapot or mug
2. Pour boiling water and cover; leave until the drink has cooled enough

3. Sweeten if required

Drink up to three times a day if required.

Day's Lovely Cayenne Pepper Ointment

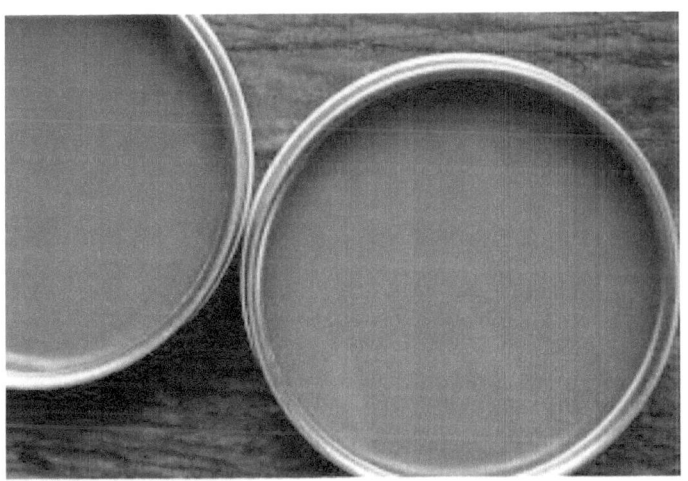

Cayenne pepper contains high amounts of capsaicin. Capsaicin was first officially discovered and extracted by Christian Friedrich Bucholz in 1816, just two short years before his death.

The medical community uses cayenne pepper and its active component **capsaicin** for a wide array of treatments but even more so as a topical analgesic that relieves pain related to shingles, diabetic neuropathy, rheumatoid arthritis, osteoarthritis, and psoriasis by desensitizing local nerves. It is also a very useful diaphoretic, which means that it promotes sweating.

The capsaicin in hot peppers stimulates blood flow, easing rheumatic, arthritic, and osteoarthritis pain. It also helps soothe sore muscles and bruising.

This Cayenne Pepper Ointment is to die for. Just lather some on your body in an area that is feeling pain and let it do its magic!

Ingredients:

- 1 tbsp cayenne pepper powder
- 5 tbsp coconut oil

Instructions:

1. Melt the oil over low heat and stir in the pepper – do not breathe the pepper powder in
2. Pour into a small jar and cool before sealing the jar
3. Use ½ tsp each time, three times a day, if needed, and wash your hands after each use. Do NOT get it into your nose or eyes.

Tremendous Turmeric Cough Syrup

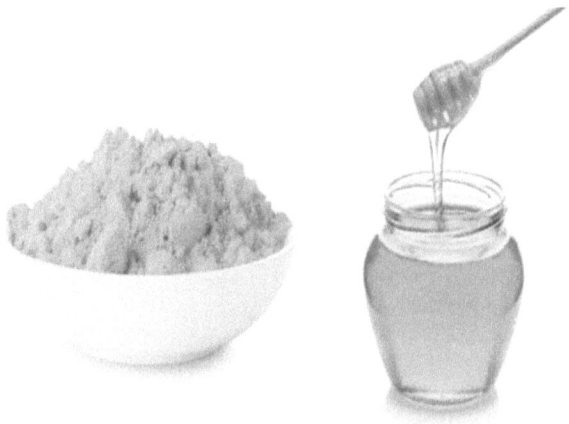

The use of **turmeric** dates back nearly 4000 years to the Vedic culture in India, where it was used as a culinary spice and had some religious significance.

It probably reached China by 700 ad, East Africa by 800 ad, West Africa by 1200 ad, and Jamaica in the eighteenth century.

Turmeric is excellent for easing inflammation from bronchitis, and honey thins mucus and eases coughing.

Use this Tremendous Turmeric Cough Syrup to sooth your sore throat and stimulate the body's natural healing processes to see that it goes away for good!

Ingredients:

- 1 tsp turmeric powder
- 8 oz. water
- 1 tbsp honey
- 1 tsp fresh squeezed lemon juice

Instructions:

1. Pour boiling water into a mug and stir the lemon, turmeric, and honey in

2. Leave to cool and drink the whole much, three times a day, on an empty stomach, for as long as needed.

Amazing Aloe-Lavender Burn Balm

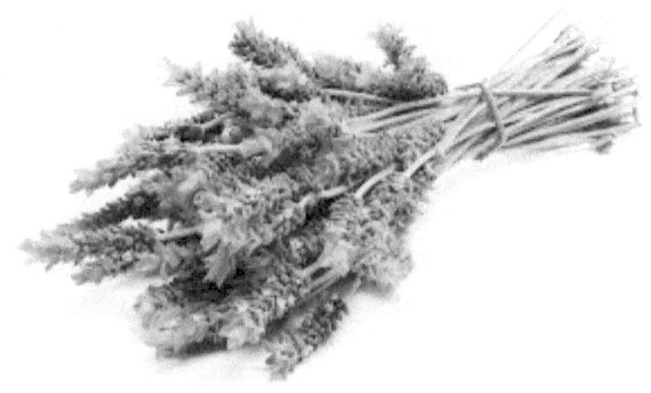

History shows us that the powerful, loving plant known as Aloe Vera is one of the oldest mentioned plants on record due to its medicinal properties and health benefits.

Ancient Chinese and Egyptians were known to have used Aloe Vera to treat burns, wounds, and reduce fever. It is also interesting to note that the Aloe Vera plant is one of the most studied herbs in the natural products category.

The Greek physician to the Roman army, Dioscorides, made note that lavender taken internally would relieve indigestion, sore throats, headaches, and externally cleaned wounds.

Beyond that, when we dig though natural medicine resources of the past, it is interesting to note that the Romans named the plant after its use in their bathing rituals ("lava" is to wash), realizing lavender isn't only relaxing, but also antiseptic.

Aloe and lavender are the perfect combination for soothing and healing burns. If you have a bad burn whip up a batch of this and apply it. You'll feel better in no time at all!

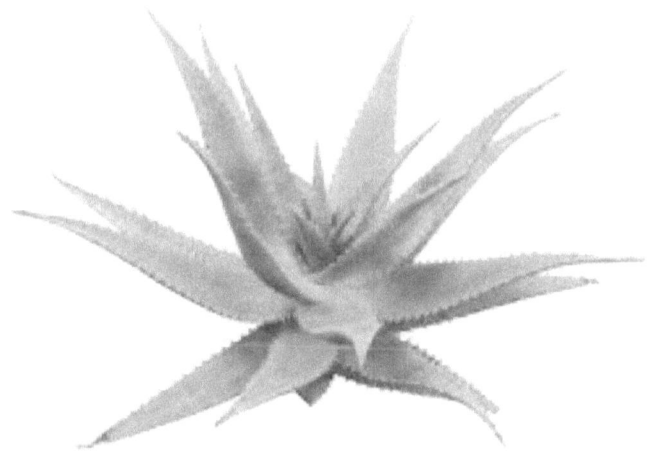

Ingredients:

- The gel from a medium aloe leaf
- 10 drops lavender essential oil

Instructions:

1. Mix the lavender and aloe gel in a bowl, blending completely
2. Apply to burns liberally and leave it to evaporate
3. Reapply as required

Stores for up to three days in the refrigerator in an airtight container.

Lucky Luscious Linden Tea

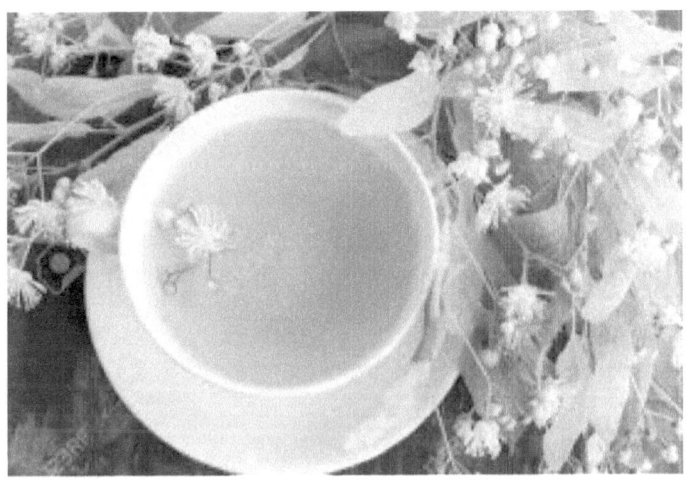

Many are unaware of this uniquely useful herb. But, in fact, Linden has been used to induce sweating for feverish colds and infections, to reduce nasal congestion, and relieve throat irritation and coughs for ages.

What makes it even more useful, is that it has sedative effects and has been used to treat nervous palpitations and high blood pressure.

But you're also not going to believe this. In addition to all the amazing different ways it has been proven in helping above, it has also been added as an ingredient in lotions due to its proven ability to relieve itchy skin.

Now, putting all that aside, this Lucky Luscious Linden Tea will calm your nerves and relieve the pent up stress in your head and body.

Go ahead and make yourself a pot, you won't believe the mood adjustment you'll see in yourself after finishing it off!

Ingredients:

- 3 cups boiling water
- 1 tbsp dried linden flowers

Instructions:

1. Using a teapot with a mesh strainer, add

the flowers to the strainer and pour the
water over

2. Cover and leave for 15 minutes
3. Sweeten as required, drink as often as you
   like.

Day's Echinacea Cold Care Herbal Tea

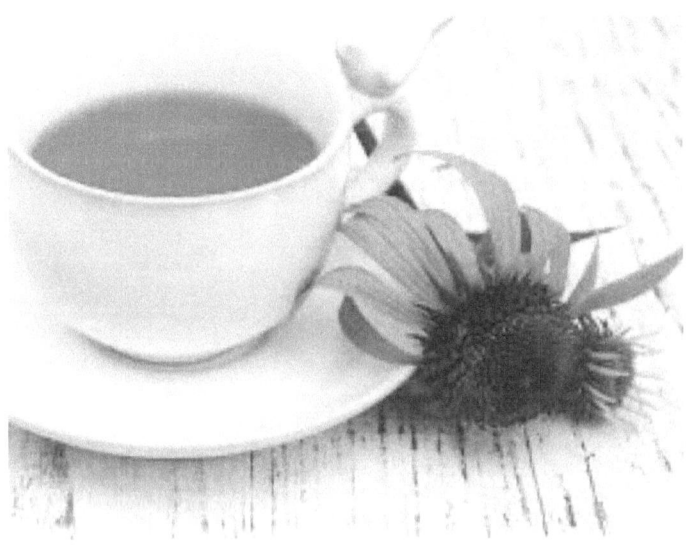

Echinacea was brought to the American health

profession in 1887 by John Uri Lloyd, a famous pharmacist and manufacturer of herbal medicines.

Later it became widely used and recommended by thousands of doctors as a very effective herbal medicine of the late 1800's and early 1900's.

Echinacea has long been used to relieve cold symptoms and blended with thyme, peppermint, and hyssop; it has the ability to reduce the symptoms of a cold quickly.

Warning: Leave the hyssop out if you are pregnant as it has been shown to cause unwanted side effects.

Consult your doctor or medical practitioner before using it if you are pregnant.

Ingredients:

- 2 oz. dried echinacea root
- 1 oz dried hyssop
- 1 oz dried peppermint
- 1 oz dried thyme
- 2 cups water for each dose
- Honey to sweeten – optional

Instructions:

1. Chop the echinacea and combine with the other herbs
2. Pour 2 cups boiling water over 2 tbsp of the mixture
3. Leave to steep for about 10 or 15 minutes, strain and sweeten if required.

Charming Chamomile Cinnamon Cough Syrup

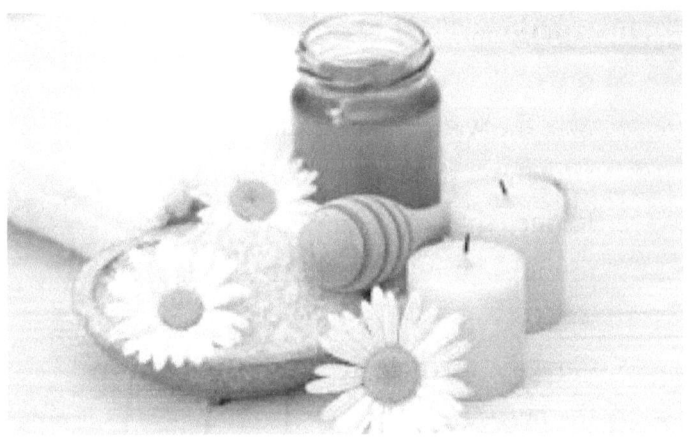

Chamomile and cinnamon both ease coughing, soothe a sore throat, and help you to rest. Using the

Charming Chamomile Cinnamon Cough Syrup to get rid of that nasty sore throat that has been bothering you all day!

Ingredients:

- 4 cups of water
- ¼ cup dried OR ½ cup fresh chamomile flowers
- ¼ cup grated ginger root
- 1 tbsp cinnamon powder
- 1 cup honey

Instructions:

1. Mix the water, chamomile, ginger, and cinnamon in a pan and bring to a boil
2. Reduce the heat, simmer for about 15 minutes, or until the mixture has reduced by 50%
3. Cool the mixture then strain to remove the herbs
4. Add the honey and heat gently, stirring to combine
5. Cool in a jar before capping and storing for up to a month in the refrigerator

6. Take 1 tbsp up to five times per day; children can have 1 tsp up to five times per day.

8. CAREFREE CALENDULA FIRST AID SALVE

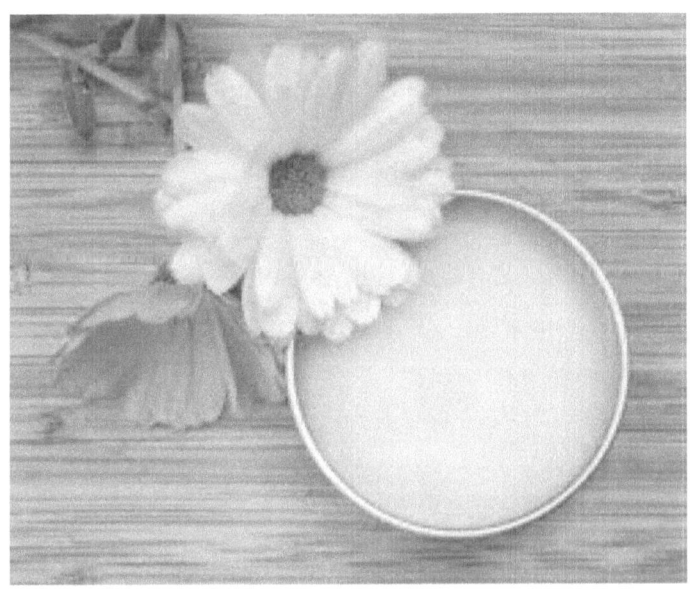

It is interesting to learn that Calendula was first

found to be growing in European gardens and that it has been used medicinally since 12th century.

Mainly, the flowers were made into extracts, tinctures, balms, salves and applied directly to skin to help heal wounds and to soothe inflamed and damaged skin.

Calendula is one of nature's antibiotics, promoting the regeneration of tissues and speeding up healing time.

With the Carefree Calendula First Aid Salve in hand you'll be able to bring back the life to old, damaged skin. Use your salve to provide some tender loving care, your skin will thank you!

Ingredients:

- 1 cup sunflower or olive oil
- 1 cup fresh OR ½ cup dried calendula flowers
- 4 tbsp beeswax, finely grated

Instructions:

1. Preheat your oven to 200°F
2. Mix the calendula and oil in an oven0safe

ceramic or glass dish and bake for between three and four hours

3. Leave it to cool and then strain to remove the flowers
4. Pour the strained oil into the dish and add the wax. Place in the warm oven and leave for a few minutes to melt the beeswax
5. Stir well and transfer to a tin or jar; cool completely and cap.
6. Apply as needed.

Flu Fighters Echinacea-Licorice Infusion

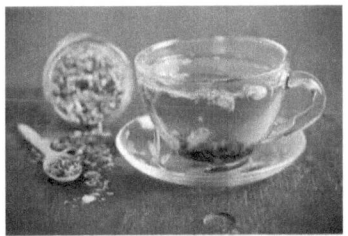

A lot of medical research has gone into this recipe. Extracts of echinacea have proven effects on the immune system, your body's defense against germs.

Research has shown that it can increase the number of white blood cells, which fight infections. A review of more than a dozen studies, published in

2014, found the herbal remedy had a very slight benefit in preventing colds.

The combination of echinacea, barberry, and licorice help fight flu symptoms effectively. The echinacea helps stop viruses, licorice coats the throat and soothes your digestive tract while barberry bark fights diarrhea.

Ingredients:

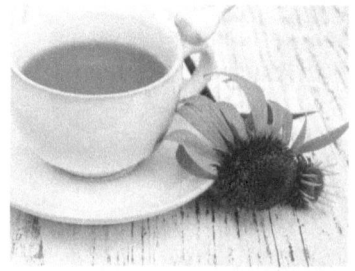

- 1-part dried barberry bark
- 1-part dried licorice root
- 1-part dried echinacea root
- 2 cups water per dose
- Honey to sweeten – optional

Instructions:

1. Mix the licorice and echinacea roots with

the barberry bark and store in a sealed container in a cool, dark place
2. When needed, add 2 cups of water to a pan with 2 tsp of the blend and bring to a boil
3. Simmer for 5 minutes and remove from the heat
4. Leave, covered, to steep for 15 minutes then strain into a mug
5. Sweeten if required
6. Drink half a cup three times a day; for children, add to their favorite juice and give them half a cup three times a day.

10. MOMMY'S MARSHMALLOW ROOT POULTICE

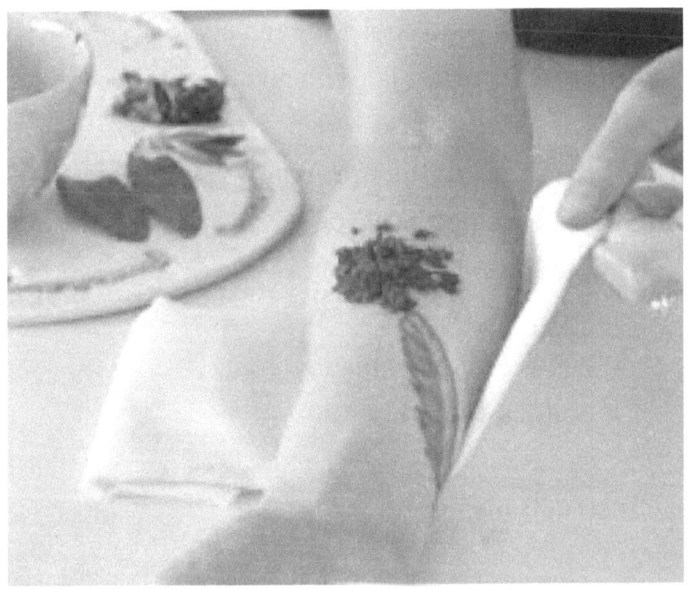

Marshmallow root has many uses in medicine, not

least the soothing properties that make it ideal as a burns poultice.

First, before getting your hands dirty so to speak, you must make sure to dry your marshmallow root:

1. Wash it thoroughly under running water
2. Chop into small pieces or grate them while they are fresh
3. Use a dehydrator it a warm oven to dry the roots
4. They are done when they are brittle and hard; leave to cool and then powder
5. Store in a glass jar with an airtight lid

Now we can begin the process of making this absolutely gorgeous poultice!

Ingredients:

- Powdered marshmallow root
- Boiling water

Instructions:

1. Put some powdered root into a glass bowl – as much as you need for the treatment

2. Add boiling water slowly, stirring until you get a paste
3. Leave to cool a bit and then apply to the burn
4. Cover with a bandage o

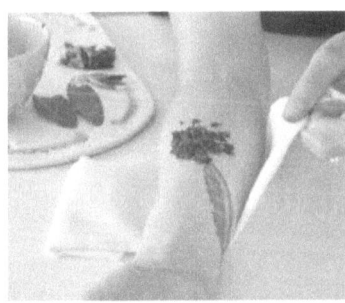

1. r a cloth.

11. COOLING PRECISION
PEPPERMINT COMPRESS

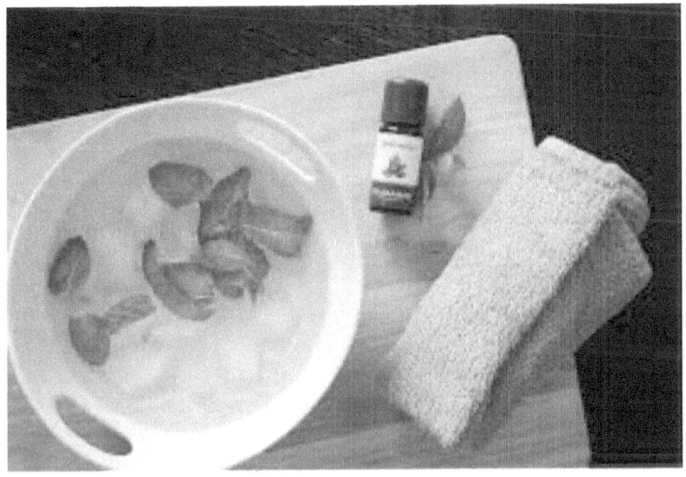

Peppermint is an herb has been used as a remedy for indigestion since Ancient Egyptian times.

Research shows that dried peppermint leaves

were found in Egyptian pyramids dating back to 1000 b.c. and possibly even further back than that.

Further evidence points to the fact that the ancient Greeks and Romans valued it as a stomach soother. In more contemporary times, peppermint was first listed in the London Pharmacopoeia in 1721.

But, all of this just brings me to my main point. Peppermint is wonderful for relieving headaches.

If you don't have any peppermint essential oil to hand, use a peppermint tea bag or steep a handful of fresh leaves in hot water to make a very effective cooling peppermint compress.

Ingredients:

- 2 peppermint teabags
- 6 ice cubes
- 2 cups boiling water
- 4-inch by 4-inc piece of cloth

Instructions:

1. Put the teabags into a bowl and add the water. Cover and leave for 20 minutes or until cool

2. Remove the tea bags, squeezing them into the bowl
3. Add the ice
4. Dip the cloth into the liquid, squeeze it out and place it over your forehead; close your eyes, and leave it. Repeat as often as needed.

The Cool Chamomile Infusion

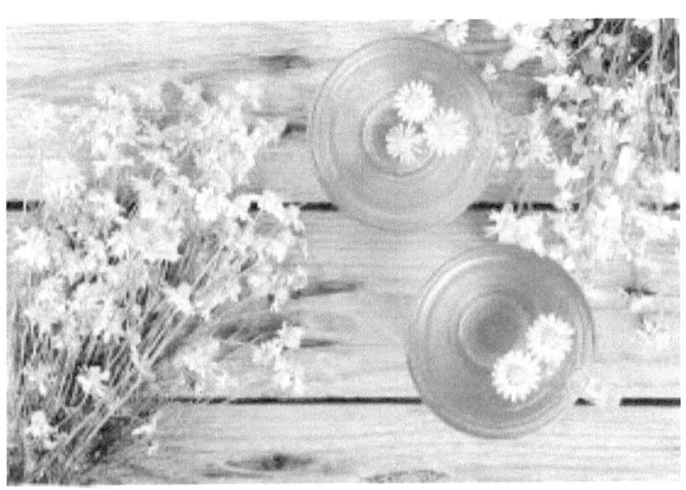

An interesting nuance that I came across while

doing my research was the similarities and differences between an infusion and a tea.

Simply put an infusion is a beverage consisting of a liquid which has had other ingredients steeped in it to extract useful qualities while tea is (uncountable) the dried leaves or buds of the tea plant.

So when we are not referring to something that uses a tea leaf or bud then we can't really call it a tea.

Chamomile is perfect for heartburn, typically brought on by indigestion or stress.

The chamomile calms you and helps with digestion, while the honey soothes the lining of your esophagus, helps digestion, and helps with healing.

Use this Cool Chamomile Infusion to relax and calm your achy nerves, reduce the stress from a long hard day at work or let it sooth your upset stomach.

Ingredients:

- 4 tbsp dried OR 2 tbsp fresh chamomile flowers
- 2 cups water
- 2 tbsp honey

Instructions:

1. Put the chamomile into a pan and add the water
2. Bring to a boil, reduce heat and simmer for about 10 to 15 minutes; the volume should reduce to about half
3. Sieve the mixture into a mug; use a spoon to press the liquid through. Add honey and stir well
4. Cool and drink as often as you need.

13. STUPENDOUS SLIPPERY ELM INFUSION

Stupendous Slippery Elm Infusion

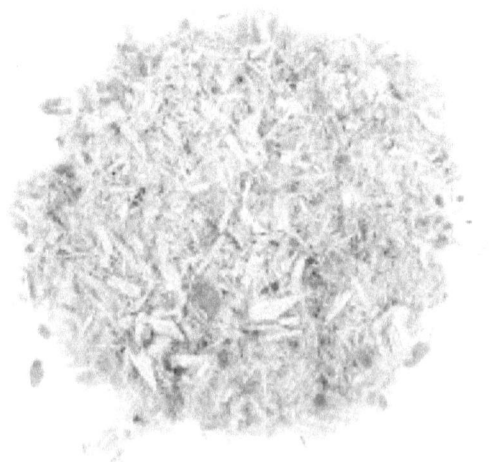

By far the Slippery Elm has one of the coolest backstories I have ever come across.

It was named after the mucilaginous inner bark which pioneers in North America chewed for quenching thirst.

Slippery Elm was official in the United States Pharmacopeia from 1820-1936 as a demulcent and used in poultices for gunshot wounds by physicians during the American Revolution.

Now, let's get to the point shall we? Slippery elm is excellent for coating the lining of your intestines and reducing inflammation.

It can prevent constipation, alleviate diarrhea, and get your bowels moving regularly; use any time you have an upset stomach.

If you have any of the tummy problems mentioned above, this Stupendous Slippery Elm Infusion is going to clear them right up!

Ingredients:

- 2 cups boiling hot water
- 1 tbsp honey
- 1 tbsp slippery elm powder
- 1 tsp fresh lemon juice

- Include other ingredients as desired

Instructions:

1. Mix all the ingredients together in the same mug
2. Leave it to steep until cool enough to drink
3. Drink one mug up to three times a day as needed.

Radical Raspberry Leaf Infusion

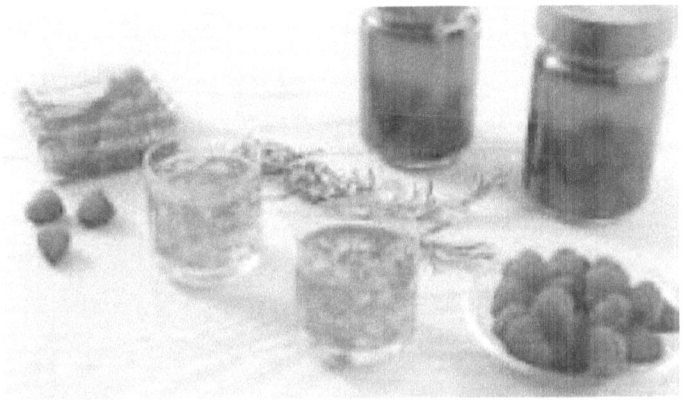

Raspberries have been enjoyed by the human race
for thousands of years. Medicinal uses of raspberries

are often found in literature, with references to raspberry leaf tea dating to the sixteenth century.

Now, in regard to its medicinal use, Raspberry leaf is commonly used as a uterine tonic. In fact, it has been recorded that as many as 25% of women in the United States use raspberry leaf during pregnancy.

What is even more interesting is that up to one-third of U.S. nurse midwives use raspberry leaf to stimulate labor in their patients. A review of the existing studies demonstrated a positive trend toward decreases in the length of first and second stage of labor and operative vaginal delivery.

Raspberry leaf is one of the best natural remedies for cramps, relaxing and easing the muscles. Use this amazing Radical Raspberry Leaf Infusion to sooth that sorry tummy and give those stomach muscles a bit of tender loving care.

Ingredients:

- 5 raspberry leaves (fresh)
- 2 cups water
- Honey for sweetening

Instructions:

1. Place the leaves into a saucepan and add the water
2. Bring to a boil and reduce the heat; leave to simmer for 10 to 15 minutes – the liquid should reduce by about 50%
3. Strain the liquid into a large mug, sweeten with honey and leave to cool slightly.

Willy's Willow Bark Muscle Rub

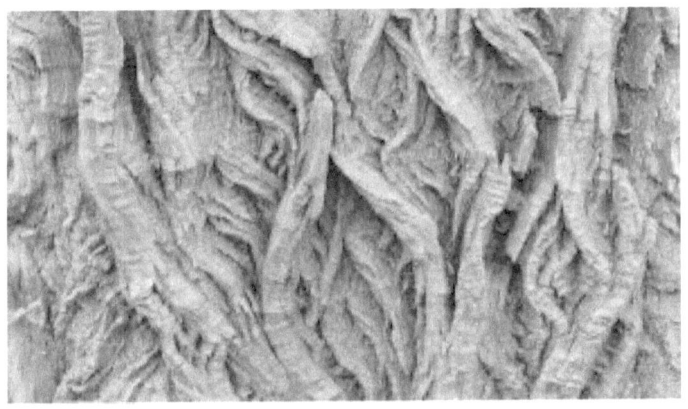

Willow bark has been found to be a useful medicinal herb for ages. The famous Greek physician Hippocrates in the fifth century BCE even recommended chewing on willow bark to relieve pain or fever and drinking tea made from it to relieve pain during childbirth.

Willow bark is not only a very effective herb in internal remedies, but it also makes a great topical remedy for sore muscles.

Use Willy's Willow Bark Muscle Rub to relax and rejuvenate your aching muscles so they can be brought back to life in your next outdoor adventure or physical exercise routine.

Ingredients:

- 1 dried habanero pepper
- 3 oz dried chopped willow bark
- ½ cup water
- 2 cups grain alcohol (95%)

Instructions:

1. Place the pepper and willow bark into a canning jar, about 1-quart, with a tight lid
2. Pour in the alcohol and the water, tighten the lid and leave in a cool dark place for 6 to 8 weeks; swirl it once a day
3. When it has cured, sieve the liquid into a

large bowl, using the back of a spoon to mash the herbs, so al the alcohol comes out

4. Transfer the liquid to a dark glass bottle, preferably with a narrow neck, and store in a dark, cool place

5. When needed, soak a cotton pad or cloth with 1 tbsp of the liquid and apply it to the sore area – keep it away from your eyes and nose.

16. CALYPSO CHAMOMILE EUCALYPTUS GARGLE

Calypso Chamomile Eucalyptus Gargle

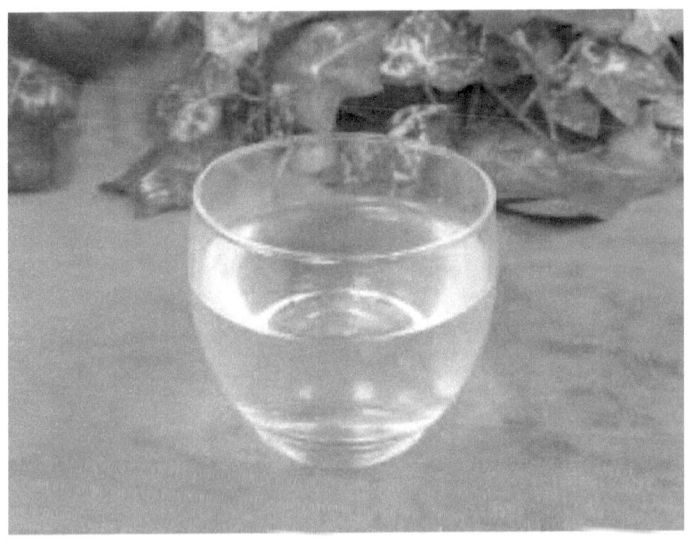

Eucalyptus oil was prominent in the Aborigines.

Touted as a cure-all medication, the eucalyptus tree was harvested and adapted by many. To this day over 700 varieties of eucalyptus exist.

Chamomile and eucalyptus are great for soothing swollen sore throats, keeping infection at bay, and shortening your illness duration.

The Calypso Chamomile Eucalyptus Gargle is an immune system booster capable of both preventing infection in the throat and mouth.

Use the gargle to fight back that sore throat and eliminate it for good. Give the gargle a chance to work its magic for you!

Ingredients:

- 2 tbsp dried OR 4 tbsp fresh chamomile flowers
- 3 drops eucalyptus oil
- 2 cups water

Instructions:

1. Put the chamomile and the water into a pan and bring to a boil
2. Turn the heat down and leave to simmer for 15 minutes

3. Sieve the mixture into a jar, using a spoon to get as much liquid as possible out of the flowers
4. Leave to cool and then add the oil. Cap the jar tightly, shake and store in the refrigerator
5. Gargle as many times as required throughout the day, using 1 to 2 tbsp of the liquid – do NOT swallow it as it may cause stomach upset.

Classy Chamomile Ice Pops

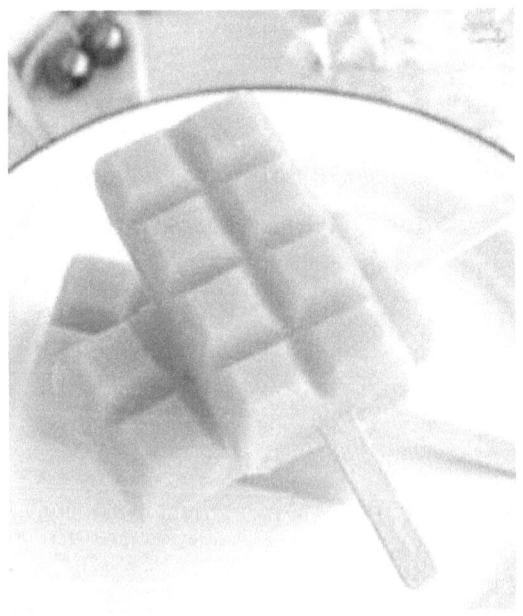

Chamomile preparations have been commonly used to heal and reduce symptoms of hay fever, inflammation, muscle spasms, menstrual disorders, insomnia, ulcers, wounds, gastrointestinal disorders, rheumatic pain, and hemorrhoids

If you have a sore tooth, a patient missing teeth or a teething baby, these ice pops can really hit the spot, helping ease pain and giving a good bout of refreshment to boot.

In fact if it's a hot summer day you have no excuse for not whipping up a brand new batch of Serena Day's Classy Chamomile Ice Pops right this moment!

Ingredients:

- 4 tbsp dried OR 8 tbsp fresh chamomile – if you don't have any use 4 chamomile teabags
- 4 cups water

Instructions:

1. Place the flowers or tea bags into a pan and add the water

2. Bring to a boil, turn the heat down and leave to simmer for about 10 or 15 minutes – the liquid should reduce by half
3. Remove from the heat and leave to cool
4. Pour into pop molds and freeze overnight

Caretaker's Calendula Infusion

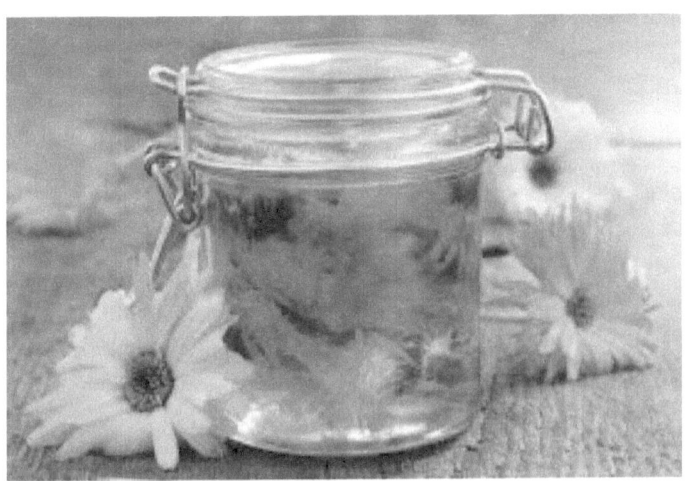

The medical research is very clear when it comes to Calendula. The verdict is that it's a highly valuable medicinal herb with a host of different healing properties.

Although there are about 12-20 species of the genus *Calendula*. Only about 4 species have been found to contain the healing power we have come to expect from nature.

Pharmacological studies reveal that *C. officinalis* exhibits antibacterial, antiviral, anti-inflammatory, anti-tumor and antioxidant properties; *C. arvensis* possesses antibacterial, anti-inflammatory, antimutagenic and hemolytic activities; and *C. suffruticosa* exhibits antimicrobial activity. *C. officinalis* has been included in number of herbal formulations, which are in clinical use for the treatment of various ailments like central nervous system disorders.

Calendula is an excellent treatment for thrush and nappy rash in children. When it comes to adults it has been proven to alleviate athlete's foot, jock itch, and ringworm.

Go ahead and whip up a pot of the **Caretaker's Calendula Infusion** today!

Ingredients:

- 6 tsp fresh OR 3 tsp dried calendula flowers
- 2 cups water

Instructions:

1. Put the water and flowers into a pan and bring to a boil
2. Reduce the heat and simmer until the liquid has reduced by half, about 10 or 15 minutes
3. Strain the mixture into a jar, using a spoon to get the liquid out of the flowers
4. Tightly cap the jar and leave to cool
5. Transfer a little to a new spray bottle and spray the infected areas. Use up to three times a day.

Serena's Sweet Dream Herbal Tea Blend

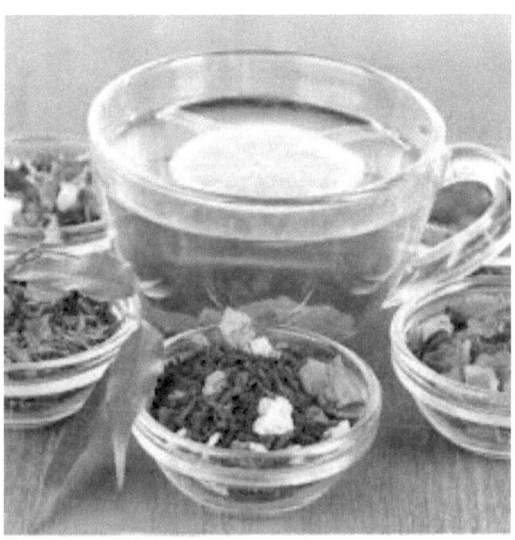

We all get insomnia from time to time. Everybody

has a day here and there that they just can't resolve in their mind when they get home.

It leaves us up late worrying and replaying what it was that put us out of our element. But, there is good news with the right herbal tea blend, we can put those racing thoughts to ease as we relax and ease the mind.

If you want to bulletproof your sleep and increase the odds of a better night's rest when you hit the hay, go ahead and whip up a pot of Serena's Sweet Dream Herbal Tea Blend.

Ingredients:

- 1 cup dried passionflower
- 1 cup dried chamomile flowers
- 1 cup chopped dried valerian root
- 1 cup dried lemon balm
- Honey to sweeten – optional

Instructions:

1. Combine the dried herbs together and store in a dark, cool place in an airtight container – this will keep for up to a year

2. Use 2 tsp of the mix per cup of boiling water
3. Leave to steep for about 15 to 20 minutes then sweeten if required
4. Drink a cup an hour before bed.

The Rosemary Rejuvenation Scalp Tonic

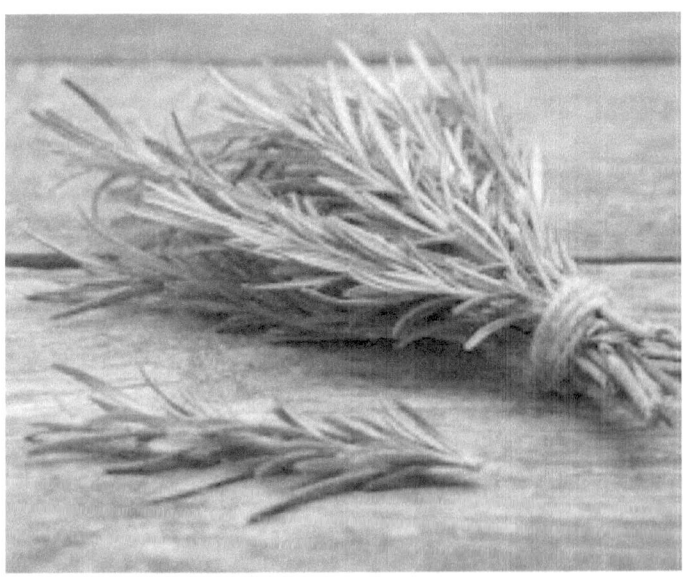

Rosemary doesn't just smell wonderful; it also has antifungal and antibacterial properties that make it great for treating dandruff. Add the borax, and you have a wonderfully natural way of clearing dandruff.

If you want to give your scalp a real treat, the Rejuvenation Scalp Tonic is what it's craving.

Ingredients:

- 1 cup fresh OR 2 cups dried rosemary, crumbled
- Cups water
- ½ cup of borax

Instructions:

1. Mix the rosemary and water in a pan and bring to the boil.
2. Reduce heat and simmer until the liquid has reduced by around 50%, about 15 to 20 minutes
3. Strain the liquid into a bowl, pressing as much liquid out of the rosemary as you can
4. Add the borax and stir, making sure it dissolves

5. Cool completely and transfer to a clean spray bottle
6. Spritz onto wet or dry hair daily, massaging into your scalp; leave for at least 30 seconds before washing out.

AFTERWORD

There's no doubt that being able to make your own medicines for common ailments will not only save you money; it will save you time in having to visit the doctor too.

Most herbs are simple to grow, and, with a little care, you can have a blooming herb garden fairly quickly – do be aware that some will take over if you let them.

The most important thing to understand is how to use your herbs safely. While you may think they are harmless – they're only plants, after all, right? – used incorrectly, and on the wrong people, they can have serious side effects.

Make sure you do your homework thoroughly, check for allergies and, where necessary, seek medical advice before you use any herbal remedies you find yourself extremely unsure of.

I hope you enjoyed my beginner's guide to herbal medicine. If you liked this guide and had fun with it, I'd like to invite you to read a few pages of my recently published guide on making all natural lotion bars.

Click on the link below to take a quick look:

20 Amazing Lotion Bars: How to Make Beautiful and Organic Lotion Bars With Ease!

Parting is always such sweet sorrow but hopefully I leave you now as a much more confident junior herbalist with an intermediate understanding of herbalism.

It is also my sincere hope that you feel better about using the effective medicinal herbs I've discussed in this guide and have the ability to make over a dozen amazing herbal remedies that you can use to help yourself, your family and your friends. Thank you so much for reading.

Sincerely,

Serena Day

ABOUT THE AUTHOR

Serena Day was born in Auckland, New Zealand in 1983. She is professional non-fiction author with a passion for creating exceptional guides centered around environmental topics, natural recipes and eco-friendly arts and crafts.

Serena's other passions include, cooking, hiking, reading and riding her Vespa around town. When it comes to her published titles, her main goal is to help her readers to live better lives through hands-on-learning and self-discovery.

Do Not Go Yet; One Last Thing To Do

If you enjoyed this book or found it useful, I'd be very grateful if you'd post a short review on Amazon. Your support really does make a difference, and I read all the reviews personally so I can get your feedback and make this book even better.

Thanks again for your support!

REFERENCES

https://www.chrysalisnaturalmedicine.com/

https://www.americanherbalistsguild.com/

https://medlineplus.gov/herbalmedicine.html

https://www.rusticfarmlife.com/

https://blog.mountainroseherbs.com/

https://theherbalacademy.com/

https://preppersunlimited.com/

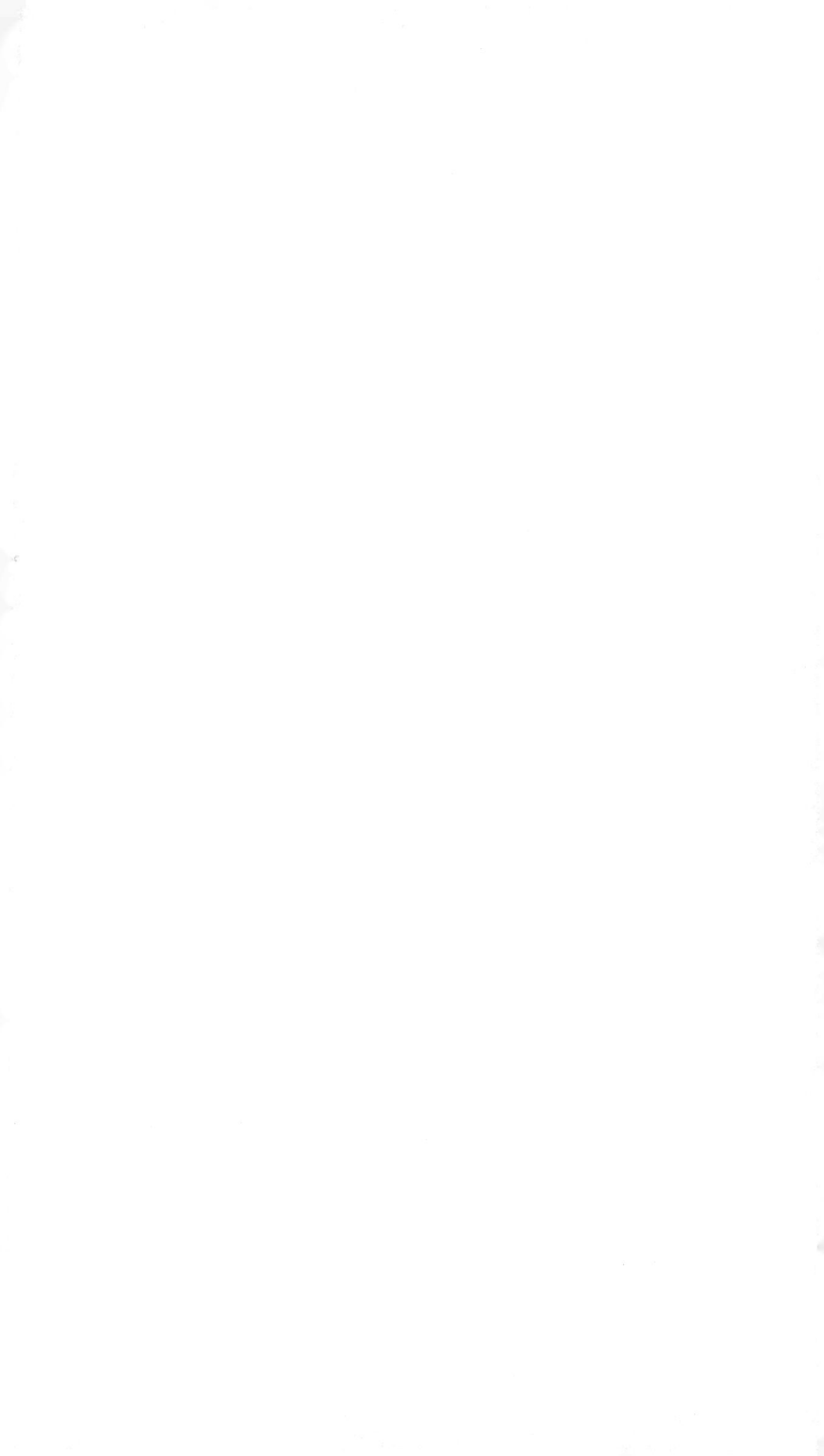

www.ingramcontent.com/pod-product-compliance
Lightning Source LLC
Chambersburg PA
CBHW030637220526
45463CB00004B/1553